Ultrasound Imaging in Acute and Chronic Kidney Disease

IRRIV
International
Renal Research
Institute Vicenza

Contributions to Nephrology

Vol. 188

Series Editor

Claudio Ronco Vicenza

Ultrasound Imaging in Acute and Chronic Kidney Disease

Volume Editors

Mario Meola Pisa
Ilaria Petrucci Pisa
Claudio Ronco Vicenza

74 figures, 58 in color, and 8 tables, 2016

KARGER Basel · Freiburg · Paris · London · New York · Chennai · New Delhi · Bangkok · Beijing · Shanghai · Tokyo · Kuala Lumpur · Singapore · Sydney

Contributions to Nephrology
(Founded 1975 by Geoffrey M. Berlyne)

Mario Meola
Department of Internal Medicine
Sant'Anna School of Advanced Studies
University of Pisa
Via Savi 10
IT–56126 Pisa (Italy)

Ilaria Petrucci
Department of Internal Medicine
Sant'Anna School of Advanced Studies
University of Pisa
Via Savi 10
IT–56126 Pisa (Italy)

Claudio Ronco
Department of Nephrology
Dialysis and Transplantation
International Renal Research Institute
(IRRIV)
San Bortolo Hospital
Viale Rodolfi 37
IT–36100 Vicenza (Italy)

Library of Congress Cataloging-in-Publication Data

Names: Meola, Mario, editor. | Petrucci, Ilaria, editor. | Ronco, C. (Claudio), 1951- editor.
Title: Ultrasound imaging in acute and chronic kidney disease / volume editors Mario Meola, Ilaria Petrucci, Claudio Ronco.
Other titles: Contributions to nephrology ; v. 188.
Description: Basel ; New York : Karger, 2016. | Series: Contributions to nephrology ; vol. 188 | Includes bibliographical references and index.
Identifiers: LCCN 2016015847| ISBN 9783318058833 (hard cover : alk. paper) | ISBN 9783318058840 (ebook)
Subjects: | MESH: Renal Insufficiency, Chronic--ultrasonography | Acute Kidney Injury--ultrasonography
Classification: LCC RC918.R4 | NLM WJ 342 | DDC 616.6/14--dc23 LC record available at https://lccn.loc.gov/2016015847

Bibliographic Indices. This publication is listed in bibliographic services, including Current Contents® and Index Medicus.

www.karger.com
Printed on acid-free and non-aging paper (ISO 9706) by Kraft Druck, Ettlingen
ISSN 0302–5144
e-ISSN 1662–2782
ISBN 978–3–318–05883–3
e-ISBN 978–3–318–05884–0

Contents

Preface

Ultrasound imaging techniques today represent a complementary yet indispensable tool in the process of diagnosis and care of kidney disease. Ultrasound machines are available in most departments of intensive care and nephrology, and their use has become a routine for clinicians directly involved in patient care rather than being procedures reserved only to experienced radiologists. The so-called '*Visual Medicine*' is becoming part of the core curriculum of several disciplines and nephrology is one of the most advanced fields in this endeavor. The evolution of ultrasound equipment into smaller and flexible devices, has further contributed to the expansion of application of sonography in the process of diagnosis. The growing demand for education and training in this area has prompted us to develop this volume, timely published by Karger, in the book series 'Contributions to Nephrology'.

New generations of physicians and nurses consider renal echography to be an expansion of their physical examination of the patient, making portable ultrasound equipment similar to what the stethoscope has been in the last century. This visionary approach requires the inclusion of visual medicine in the core curriculum of young physicians and nurses to make them acquainted with the newest techniques and the potential of the imaging approach to diagnosis.

Nephrology is a subspecialty of medicine that will gather specific advantages from the wide application of ultrasound diagnostic techniques. The kidney is a deep organ in the abdomen and physical examination is often frustrating, if not useless, for the diagnosis of kidney problems. Echography has already demonstrated in recent years the enormous advantages for interventional practices such as kidney biopsy. Today, with the addition of Doppler techniques, US imaging in nephrology has further enhanced its importance.

Sonography is also important in the case of acute kidney diseases, allowing to expand the spectrum of diagnostic criteria and to trigger specific treatment strategies as in the case of acute urinary tract obstruction. The possibility to determine morphological parameters and at the same time to explore functional aspects with contrast-enhanced or Doppler ultrasound techniques, is of great value in acutely ill patients especially in the case of oliguria. The non-invasive nature of the technique and the possibility to perform a morphological analysis without potentially toxic contrast media makes echography a technique of choice in patients at risk for acute kidney injury. Recently, further improvement has been achieved in contrast-enhanced ultrasound using non-toxic gas microbubbles as the image contrast enhancer. Another advantage of modern echography is the light weight of equipment, the easy transportability and the possibility to perform examinations at the bedside without the need of transporting the patient to radiologic departments or special imaging areas of the hospital.

Of course the wide application of echography in nephrology and critical care nephrology will require an investment in equipment and education of physicians and nurses. It remains obvious that ultrasound will be a first-line approach for diagnosis while more sophisticated approaches and other imaging techniques will always require an experienced radiologist and large and expensive equipment. Nevertheless, the wider application of ultrasound techniques in clinical routine will allow to rule out at a first glance some important pathological conditions and to concentrate on an accurate diagnosis of the patient. Clinical and biochemical data should also corroborate the diagnostic pathway. Because the outcome of sonography is operator-dependent, special attention should be made to make as many specialists in the area of nephrology and intensive care acquainted with the technique. For this reason, we feel that this book may represent an important resource both for beginners and for advanced users of echography that will focus on their daily practice on diagnosis of kidney disease supported by ultrasound imaging techniques.

Mario Meola, Pisa
Ilaria Petrucci, Pisa
Claudio Ronco, Vicenza

Meola M, Petrucci I, Ronco C (eds): Ultrasound Imaging in Acute and Chronic Kidney Disease.
Contrib Nephrol. Basel, Karger, 2016, vol 188, pp 1–10 (DOI: 10.1159/000445460)

Pathophysiology and Clinical Work-Up of Acute Kidney Injury

Mario Meola[a, b] · Federico Nalesso[c] · Ilaria Petrucci[a, b] · Sara Samoni[a, c] · Claudio Ronco[c]

[a]Sant'Anna School of Advanced Studies, Pisa, [b]Department of Internal Medicine, University of Pisa, Pisa, and [c]Department of Nephrology Dialysis and Transplantation, International Renal Research Institute (IRRIV), San Bortolo Hospital, Vicenza, Italy

Abstract

Acute kidney injury (AKI), also known in the past as acute renal failure, is a syndrome characterized by the rapid loss of kidney excretory function. It is usually diagnosed by the accumulation of end products of nitrogen metabolism (urea and creatinine) or decreased urine output or both. AKI is the clinical consequence of several disorders that acutely affect the kidney, causing electrolytes and acid–base imbalance, hyperhydration and loss of depurative function. AKI is common in critical care patients in whom it is often secondary to extrarenal events. No specific therapies can attenuate AKI or accelerate renal function recovery; thus, the only treatment is supportive. New diagnostic techniques such as renal biomarkers might improve early diagnosis. Also ultrasonography helps nephrologists in AKI diagnosis, in order to describe and follow kidney alterations and find possible causes of AKI. Renal replacement therapy is a life-saving treatment if AKI is severe. If patients survive to AKI, and did not have previous chronic kidney disease (CKD), they typically recover to dialysis independence. However, evidence suggests that patients who have had AKI are at increased risk of subsequent CKD.

Definitions

The definition of acute renal failure (ARF) is usually used to describe a syndrome in which the rapid fall of glomerular filtration rate (GFR) determines retention of nitrogen catabolites with water and electrolyte imbalance and alteration in acid–base status. Loss of GFR leads to a rapid increase in serum

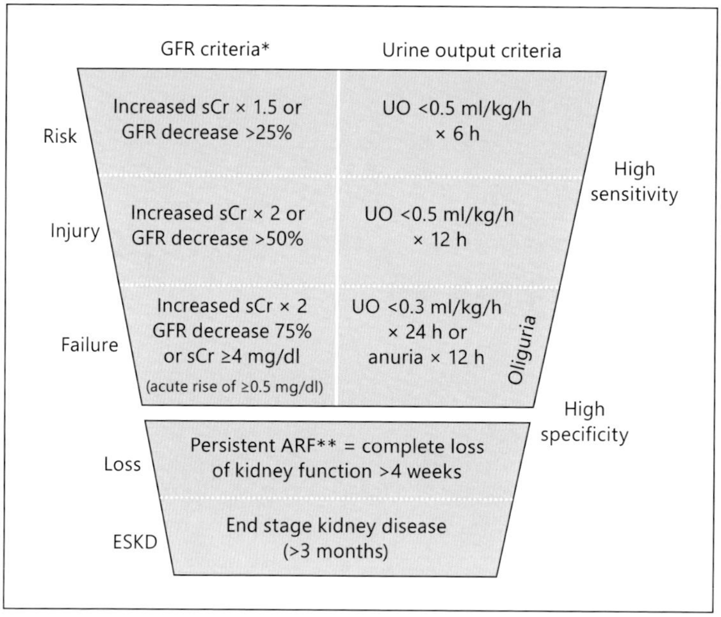

Fig. 1. Acute kidney disease: RIFLE criteria. UO = Urine output; ESRD = end stage renal disease [3].

creatinine (sCr) and may be associated with normal urine output, oliguria (urine output <500 ml/day) or anuria (urine output <100 ml/day).

Symptoms that accompany ARF vary from multi-organ failure (MOF) to acute pulmonary edema and hyperkalemia [1]. This definition has 2 limits: (1) it lacks a GFR reduction cutoff, which is needed to determine ARF and (2) sCr is not a reliable marker of GFR in hemodynamically unstable patients. In the last decade, in order to achieve a unique definition of ARF, several groups developed new criteria for ARF diagnosis. In 2004, the Acute Dialysis Quality Initiative proposed the RIFLE criteria, based on sCr and diuresis, establishing for the first time the guidelines for the treatment and prevention of ARF (fig. 1) [1–3]. RIFLE is the acronym of Risk, Injury, Failure, Loss and End-stage kidney disease, and it seems to be a good outcome predictor, showing a progressive increase in mortality as RIFLE class increases.

In 2007, the Acute Kidney Injury Network (AKIN) introduced a modified version of the RIFLE classification, in order to increase the sensitivity and specificity of AKI diagnosis. The AKIN classification (fig. 2) states that AKI diagnosis must be considered only after achieving an adequate hydration status and after excluding urinary obstruction. AKIN classification relies only on sCr and not on GFR changes; baseline sCr is unnecessary in the AKIN classification, and it requires at least 2 values of sCr within a period of 48 hours. AKI is defined by

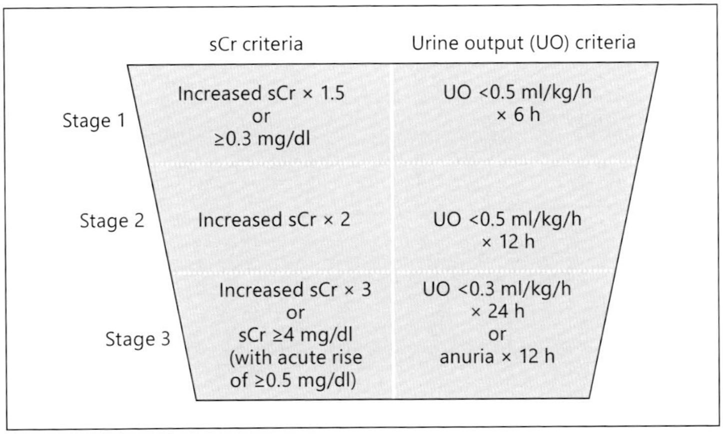

Fig. 2. Stages of acute kidney disease according to the akin group. AKIN considers the same variations of sCr as reported in RIFLE criteria, but an increased sCr of 0.3 mg/dl in 48 h is also considered as a sign of AKI [14].

the sudden decrease of renal function in 48 h, defined by an increase in absolute sCr of at least 0.3 mg/dl or by a percentage increase in sCr >50% (1.5 × baseline value) or by a decrease in the urine output (documented oliguria <0.5 ml/kg/h for >6 h). AKIN classification, as RIFLE, allowed the identification and stratification of AKI in most hospitalized patients and was independently associated with their outcome.

In 2012, the new Kidney Disease Improving Global Outcome (KDIGO) classification for AKI has been published. In KDIGO guidelines, AKI is defined as any of the following:

- increase in sCr by ≥0.3 mg/dl (≥26.5 mmol/l) within 48 h; or
- increase in sCr ≥1.5 times baseline, which is known or presumed to have occurred within the prior 7 days; or
- urine volume <0.5 ml/kg/h for 6 h.

AKI severity is staged according to the criteria as shown in table 1. The cause of AKI should be determined whenever possible.

Etiology

AKI is a broad clinical syndrome that includes different causes, such as specific kidney diseases (acute interstitial nephritis, acute glomerular and vasculitic renal diseases), non-specific conditions (ischemia, toxic and/or drug injury), as well as extrarenal pathologies (pre-renal damage and acute post-renal obstructive nephropathy). More conditions may coexist in the same patient,

Table 1. KDIGO criteria for AKI staging

Stage	sCr	Urine output
1	1.5–1.9 times baseline OR ≥0.3 mg/dl (≥26.5 mmol/l) increase	<0.5 ml/kg/h for 6–12 h
2	2.0–2.9 times baseline	<0.5 ml/kg/h for ×12 h for ≥12 h
3	3.0 times baseline OR Increase in sCr to ≥4.0 mg/dl (≥353.6 mmol/l) OR Initiation of renal replacement therapy OR In patients <18 years, decrease in eGFR to <35 ml/min per 1.73 m^2	<0.3 ml/kg/h for ≥24 h OR Anuria for ≥12 h

and moreover, epidemiological evidence supports that even mild, reversible AKI has important clinical consequences, including increased risk of death [4, 5].

Although AKI can be determined by different causes, nephron injury is always due to an important discrepancy between oxygen and nutrients demand and availability. Usually, AKI causes are divided into pre-renal, renal and post-renal. The prevalence of each clinical type is not well known and varies according to the criteria of classification used. Pre-renal AKI represents 50–60% of cases and it is due to a sudden decrease in renal perfusion with reduced GFR. Hypotension (systolic blood pressure <80 mm Hg and diastolic blood pressure <60 mm Hg) or shock may be consequent to different conditions such as hypovolemia due to excessive fluid loss (bleeding, diarrhea/vomiting, severe burns, diuretic abuse), insufficient fluid intake, pump defect (acute or chronic heart failure) or, lastly, to excessive vasodilation (sepsis, anaphylaxis, iatrogenic causes). In these cases, renal parenchyma is not damaged if volemia, and consequently GFR, is rapidly recovered. In other words, pre-renal AKI is a functional reversible status if it is quickly treated.

Parenchymal causes of AKI are ischemia, primitive glomerular and interstitial diseases. Drugs or toxic substances are the most common causes of AKI, due to their concentration into tubular cells and interstitial space. Acute injury may overlap with pre-existing chronic kidney disease (CKD), so AKI becomes a major cause of damage progression toward CKD stage 5. In critical care units, AKI is almost associated with MOF and sepsis.

Post-renal causes of AKI are all conditions that determine urinary tract obstruction, which can be intraluminal lithiasis or clots, urothelial cancer,

Table 2. Physiopathology of acute kidney damage

Microvascular		Tubular
glomerular	medullary	
↑ Vasoconstriction	↓ O_2 →	Cytoskeletal breakdown Loss of polarity
↓ Vasodilation		Apoptosis and necrosis
↑ Endothelial and vascular smooth muscle cellular damage	Inflammatory vasoactive mediators	Desquamation of viable and necrotic cells Tubular obstruction
↑ Leukocyte endothelial adhesion	←	Back-leak

Summary of the complex interactions between microcirculation and renal tubule that cause acute kidney damage. PGE2 = Prostaglandin E_2.

retroperitoneal fibrosis or tumors, bladder diseases, prostate and/or urethral obstructions. Post-renal AKI is a reversible condition when obstructive causes are removed.

Pathogenesis

Acute tubular damage is due to a complex sequence of events, which varies depending on the specific etiology of the syndrome. However, a final common pathway correlated to segmental or widespread kidney ischemia characterizes pathophysiological processes that lead to injury and organ dysfunction. Table 2 summarizes the complex interactions between microcirculation and renal tubule on which organ dysfunction is based [6]. The first step of AKI is an important vasoconstriction due to increased concentrations of angiotensin II and endothelin I and to hyperactivity of the sympathetic system. Vasoconstriction is moreover enhanced by a reduced availability of vasodilators such as nitric oxide, acetylcholine and bradykinin. These factors induce endothelial dysfunction, increase leukocyte adhesiveness and activate the coagulation cascade. The final result is a diffused small vessels thrombosis with enhanced leukocyte activation, inflammation and release of cytokines. The reduced availability of oxygen induces the tubular epithelial cell damage and the release of further proinflammatory mediators. In other words, damage progression is based on tubular epithelial cell damage. In fact, ischemic or toxic tubular epithelium injury determines a rapid loss of cell polarity and of the cytoskeleton structural integrity. These factors lead to tubular epithelium collapse, to loss of adhesion molecules and membrane proteins, and then to apoptosis and cell necrosis. If the injury is severe, the basement membrane looses the epithelial layer; so there is an exfoliation of tubular cells into the tubular lumen. Exfoliated tubular cells get mixed with debris and tubular proteins (Tamm–Horsfall protein and fibronectin); thus determining the formation of cylinders that obstruct the lumen and increase intratubular pressure. The decrease of GFR and the presence of urine back-filtration into the interstitial space are a direct consequence of the increased intratubular pressure. Moreover, vasoactive agents and pro-inflammatory mediators released from activated tubular cells determine an autocrine and paracrine action on tubular cells and on microcirculation, amplifying the effects of inflammation and vasoconstriction. So, inflammation mainly contributes to the sequence of events leading to acute tubular necrosis (ATN) [7]. Unlike the heart and brain, the kidneys can repair ischemic or toxic injury. It seems that a subpopulation of stem cells localized into the interstitium or into the renal tubule may play a role in this recovery process. During the recovery phase, it was observed that an intense migration of epithelial cells progressively repair the areas of uncovered basement membrane until the recovery of the anatomical and functional integrity of the nephron [8].

Vascular Reactivity

The pivotal role of microcirculation in AKI pathophysiology is outlined by resistance index variations, measured by ultrasonography (US). Renal injury causes persistent vasoconstriction in two microvascular sections, that is, the pre-glomerular and the outer medulla networks [9]. In the first section, the inadequate sodium reabsorption in the proximal tubule and, thus its increased load in the distal tubule favor vasoconstriction. Vasoconstriction may persist for several hours after the injury in the outer part of the medulla causing a significant reduction in the blood flow. In this area, the low pressure of peri-tubular capillaries favors epithelial damage, leukocyte adhesion, inflammation and activation of the coagulation cascade, thus determining thrombosis of the microcirculation. Flow reduction of renal outer medullary microcirculation has negative effects on tubular cells because it further reduces the oxygen availability in this section due to the vasa recta countercurrent exchange mechanism [10]. In AKI, renal microcirculation is hyper-responsive to vasoconstrictors, hypo-responsive to vasodilators and inappropriately responsive to drops of blood perfusion pressure. During kidney ischemia, the most important vasoconstrictors are endothelin-1, angiotensin II, thromboxane A2, prostaglandin H2, leukotriene C4 and D4, adenosine and hyperactivity of the sympathetic

Table 3. Prevalence of AKI clinical forms in general population

Cause of AKI	% of patients with AKI
Pre-renal failure secondary to acute hypoperfusion	55–60
Renal failure secondary to acute parenchymal diseases	35–40
Vascular diseases of main vessels	
Renal microcirculation damage	
Ischemic or toxic acute tubular damage*	
Acute tubulointerstitial damage	
Post-renal failure secondary to urinary tract obstruction	5

* Responsible for 90% of cases of parenchymal AKI.

system [9]. Experimental data demonstrate that increased reactivity to vasoconstrictors is not limited to acute ischemic phase but can persist even several weeks after renal recovery.

Clinical and Diagnostic Problems

Clinical course, treatment and prognosis of AKI substantially differ depending on pathogenetic factors. For these reasons, etiologic diagnosis is not always easy but it is pivotal [11]. In any case, prognosis depends on the severity and duration of renal impairment, the presence/absence of underlying disorders and patient's basal conditions. The prevalence of AKI clinical forms shown in table 3 radically changes if we consider patients referred to emergency medicine and needing for temporary renal replacement therapy, ATN being the most prevalent form of AKI in these patients [12]. Several clinical data (history, body weight and blood pressure, central venous pressure, edema, jugular turgor, pulmonary stasis, uremic signs), biochemical and urinary tests (blood urea nitrogen, sCr, Na^+, K^+, Ca^{2+}, HCO_3^-, Cl^-, PO_4^{3-}, total serum protein, hemoglobin, urine specific gravity and density, cylinders, urinary excretion and fractional excretion of Na^+), morphological parameters (US, CT, MRI, renal scintigraphy) and histological features are needed to perform a differential diagnosis between the different forms of AKI.

Clinical Evaluation

AKI work-up needs an accurate medical history; so it must be carefully collected from the patient himself or from family members in case of unconscious patients. Medical history commonly allows correlating AKI with a pre-existent clinical

Table 4. Examples of urine findings according to causes of ARF

Condition	Urine osmolality (mOsm/kg)	Sodium concentration (mmol/l)	Fractional excretion of sodium (%)
Prerenal failure	>500	<20	<1
Parenchymal renal failure			
Tubular necrosis*	<350	>40	>1
Acute interstitial nephritis	<350	>40	>1
Acute glomerulonephritis**	>500	<20	<1
Post-renal failure***	<350	>40	>1

* In non-oliguric ARF due to sepsis or radiocontrast agents, the initial fractional excretion of sodium can be >1%. ** When tubulointerstitial abnormalities are associated with glomerular lesions, urine osmolality is <350 mOsm/kg and the fractional excretion of sodium is >1%. *** The fractional excretion of sodium can be <1% early in the course of obstruction (before tubular injury occurred).

condition or associating it to drugs or toxic substances. Case history allows including symptoms in a clinical scenario that can be related to initial sepsis, blood transfusion, abortion and hemolytic crisis. Finally, if clinical history reveals poisoning or use of nephrotoxic drugs, there is a very strong possibility that oliguria may be due to a toxic ATN. On the other hand, after a crush injury, it is frequent to diagnose AKI associated with crush syndrome. On this basis, patients with AKI need a multidisciplinary approach, in which each specialist gives his own contribution in order to reach the correct clinical diagnosis and to provide the best therapy.

Urine Test

Urine analysis is useful in AKI differential diagnosis. Pigmented granular casts are typical in ischemic or toxic AKI, while microscopic hematuria with dysmorphic and fragmented erythrocytes is common in acute glomerulonephritis. Patients with glomerulonephritis often show nephrotic/non-nephrotic proteinuria. On the contrary, proteinuria is low (<1 g/day) or absent in all other forms of AKI, indicating a tubular proteinuria. Some urinary parameters (osmolarity, Na^+ urinary concentration and fractional excretion of Na^+) distinguish pre-renal AKI from ATN (table 4) [13]. In fact, in pre-renal syndrome, sodium tubular reabsorption and urine concentrating capacity are preserved, while they are compromised in ATN. Patients with pre-renal AKI have a low urinary sodium concentration (<20 mmol/l) and high urine osmolality (>500 mOsm/kg). On the contrary, patients with ATN have high urinary sodium concentration (>40 mmol/l) and low urinary osmolarity (<350 mOsm/kg).

Percutaneous Renal Biopsy

Percutaneous renal biopsy (PRB) should be performed when pre- and post-renal causes of AKI have been excluded and parenchymal damage can be assessed only by histology. PRB is not indicated when AKI is superimposed to CKD, since histological results often would not guide therapeutic decisions. On the contrary, PRB is useful if a glomerular disease that could respond to a specific therapy is suspected (i.e., rapidly progressive glomerulonephritis, Goodpasture's syndrome, renal disease secondary to collagenopathy, vasculitis, hemolytic uremic syndrome, allergic interstitial nephritis and acute transplant rejection). Moreover, glomerulonephritis can be easily distinguished from an interstitial nephritis using immunofluorescence. Diffuse or focal glomerulonephrities are characterized by the nature of glomerular and basement membrane injury and by the morphology of immune complex deposits. Interstitial nephritis secondary to drugs, hyperuricemia or bacterial infections (Streptococcus, Legionella etc.) are characterized by interstitial edema and diffuse lymphocytes, plasma cells and histiocytes infiltration.

Imaging

Kidneys imaging can provide useful information in the evaluation and management of AKI. At present, several imaging modalities are used to obtain information on kidneys anatomy, to exclude obstruction, to differentiate AKI from CKD and to assess renal blood flow and GFR. US is the most widespread imaging modality used in the first level work-up of AKI, whereas the use of CT and MRI is limited by contrast agents toxicity.

Conclusion

Clinical setting of AKI is still an important challenge for nephrologists and intensivists. Histological and biochemical advances have improved our understanding on pathophysiological processes in AKI and on the recovery of kidney function after the injury. All this processes represent some potential therapeutic targets. Markers such as sCr slowly vary over time following kidney injury. For this reason, improved methods for evaluating GFR and a more rapid assessment of renal injury are likely to improve the ability to diagnose AKI earlier and to identify its clinical course more accurately. The use of biomarkers and the assessment of renal microcirculation damage with non-invasive and non-toxic imaging techniques may represent a useful tool in the diagnosis and therapeutic work-up of AKI.

References

1 Ostermann M, Chang RW: Acute kidney injury in the intensive care unit according to RIFLE. Crit Care Med 2007;35:1837–1843; quiz 1852.
2 Ronco C, Kellum JA, Bellomo R, Mehta RL: Acute dialysis quality initiative (ADQI). Nephrol Dial Transplant 2001;16:1555–1558.
3 Bellomo R, Ronco C, Kellum JA, Mehta RL, Palevsky P; Acute Dialysis Quality Initiative Workgroup: Acute renal failure – definition, outcome measures, animal models, fluid therapy and information technology needs: the second international consensus conference of the acute dialysis quality initiative (ADQI) group. Crit Care 2004;8:R204–R212.
4 Hoste EA, Clermont G, Kersten A, et al: RIFLE criteria for acute kidney injury are associated with hospital mortality in critically ill patients: a cohort analysis. Crit Care 2006; 10:R73.
5 Uchino S, Bellomo R, Goldsmith D, et al: An assessment of the RIFLE criteria for acute renal failure in hospitalized patients. Crit Care Med 2006;34:1913–1917.
6 Bonventre JV, Zuk A: Ischemic acute renal failure: an inflammatory disease? Kidney Int 2004;66:480–485.
7 Bonventre JV: Dedifferentiation and proliferation of surviving epithelial cells in acute renal failure. J Am Soc Nephrol 2003; 14(suppl 1):S55–S61.
8 Schrier RW, Wang W: Acute renal failure and sepsis. N Engl J Med 2004;351:159–169.
9 Basile DP, Donohoe DL, Phillips SA, Frisbee JC: Enhanced skeletal muscle arteriolar reactivity to ANG II after recovery from ischemic acute renal failure. Am J Physiol Regul Integr Comp Physiol 2005;289:R1770–R1776.
10 Bonventre JV: Molecular and genetic aspects of ischemic acute kidney injury; in Mount DB, Pollack M (eds): Molecular and Genetic Basis of Renal Disease: A Companion to Brenner and Rector's The Kidney. Philadelphia, Saunders Publishing, 2008, pp 531–555.
11 Singbartl K, Kellum JA: AKI in the ICU: definition, epidemiology, risk stratification, and outcomes. Kidney Int 2012;81:819–825.
12 Liaño F, Pascual J: Epidemiology of acute renal failure: a prospective, multicenter, community-based study. Madrid acute renal failure study group. Kidney Int 1996;50: 811–818.
13 Thadhani R, Pascual M, Bonventre JV: Acute renal failure. N Engl J Med 1996;334:1448–1460.
14 Mehta RL, Kellum JA, Shah SV, Molitoris BA, Ronco C, Warnock DG, Levin A: Acute Kidney Injury Network: report of an initiative to improve outcomes in acute kidney injury. Crit Care 2007;11:R31.

Claudio Ronco, MD
Department of Nephrology Dialysis and Transplantation
International Renal Research Institute (IRRIV), San Bortolo Hospital
Viale Rodolfi 37, IT–36100 Vicenza (Italy)
E-Mail cronco@goldnet.it

Meola M, Petrucci I, Ronco C (eds): Ultrasound Imaging in Acute and Chronic Kidney Disease.
Contrib Nephrol. Basel, Karger, 2016, vol 188, pp 11–20 (DOI: 10.1159/000445461)

Ultrasound in Acute Kidney Disease

Mario Meola[a, b] · Federico Nalesso[c] · Ilaria Petrucci[a, b] ·
Sara Samoni[a, c] · Claudio Ronco[c]

[a]Sant'Anna School of Advanced Studies, Pisa, [b]Department of Internal Medicine, University of Pisa, Pisa, and [c]Department of Nephrology Dialysis and Transplantation, International Renal Research Institute (IRRIV), San Bortolo Hospital, Vicenza, Italy

Abstract

Kidneys' imaging provides useful information in acute kidney injury (AKI) diagnosis and management. Today, several imaging techniques give information on kidneys anatomy, urinary obstruction, differential diagnosis between AKI and chronic kidney disease (CKD), renal blood flow and glomerular filtration rate. Ultrasound is a safe, non-invasive and repeatable imaging technique so it is widely used in the first level work-up of AKI. The utility of contrast-enhanced computed tomography and magnetic resonance imaging in AKI or in AKI during CKD is limited because of renal toxicity associated with contrast agents used.

Introduction

Technological advances in ultrasound (US) imaging have improved the possibility of characterizing tissue damage. Nevertheless, renal parenchymal diseases cannot be differentiated with US. US information originating from stationary structures or red blood cells moving into vessels can be visualized with different imaging modalities. Conventional B-Mode US provides anatomic information based on differences in acoustic impedance. Gray-scale US represents structural echoes as brightness points. Based on the Doppler effect, vascular scattering can be represented as spectral wave velocity depending on time (velocity/time curve), or as dual-scale color mapping depending on the changes in average blood velocity. The flow-in is depicted in red and the flow-out in blue. The analysis of vascular scattering enhanced by infusion of contrast agents is the basis of contrast-enhanced harmonic imaging. Perfusion pattern of tissues allows the differential diagnosis of expansive lesions. Tissue strain analysis provides a new dimension of diagnostic information. It is used in elastographic imaging to describe relative physical tissue stiffness properties. Tissue stiffness information is independent from the acoustic impedance information provided by B-Mode imaging as well as the vascular flow information provided by Doppler imaging. Adjacent tissue elements may appear identical using conventional B-Mode or Doppler imaging. When stress is applied to tissues, they show different degrees of deformation. Comparing the baseline and stress image information, each tissue element may be labeled by its relative stiffness. A lighter shade indicates relatively soft tissue (elastic), while a darker shade indicates relatively stiff tissue (non-elastic).

All these US applications may characterize the tissue damage, but the presence of artifacts and the difficulty in signal analysis do not allow a reliable diagnosis of parenchymal injury. In fact, conventional US parameters (renal diameter, parenchymal echogenicity and thickness, urinary tract status) allow a correct diagnosis in only 50–70% of acute kidney injury (AKI) and chronic kidney diseases (CKD). Doppler analysis can only provide indirect information on parenchymal microcirculation. Contrast-enhanced ultrasound (CEUS) with second generation contrast media is not very diffused in Nephrology, so diagnostic potentialities of this application in district perfusion characterization have to be verified. Finally, elastosonography applications in native kidneys are limited by organ depth but they could have a role in transplanted kidney. In conclusion, US is not always able to define kidney damage in native and in transplanted kidney, thus to define it nephrologists must still perform percutaneous renal biopsy (PRB). In any case, US is a disposable, safe and useful technique in evaluating patients with AKI or obstruction of the urinary tract in order to assess clinical work-up.

Conventional B-Mode Ultrasound

Conventional B-Mode (Brightness mode) US is the first technique for evaluating AKI and CKD patients. It is easily accessible for nephrologists and intensivists, free of complications and well tolerated. Moreover, B-Mode US can be performed at the bedside, thus determining a significant advantage, especially for critical care patients. Recent advances in digital technology and, particularly, in tissue harmonic imaging, have improved the ability to characterize kidneys' structure. Nevertheless, kidneys' structure is abnormal only in 10% of cases of

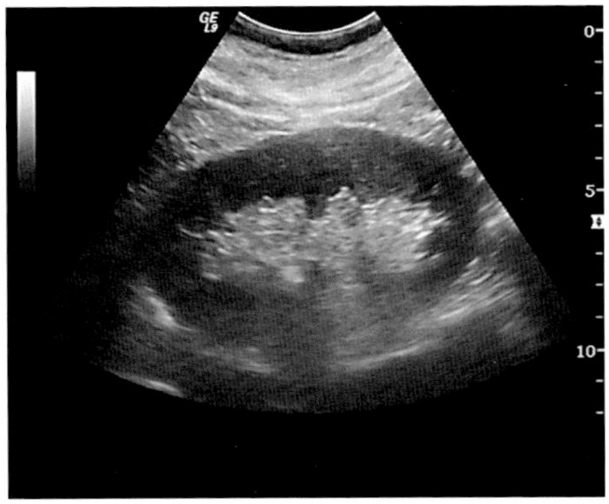

Fig. 1. Normal kidney. Grayscale B-Mode US analyzes the following parameters: 1) longitudinal diameter; 2) parenchymal thickness; 3) echogenicity; 4) profiles; 5) urinary tract status.

AKI [1]. Basic principles of B-Mode imaging are almost the same today as they were several decades ago. In B-Mode, small US pulses are sent from a transducer into the body. As the ultrasound waves penetrate body tissues some of them are reflected back to the transducer while some of them continue to penetrate deeper. The different tissues acoustic impedances along US transmission wave determine echo signals with different intensities. Echo signals from many sequential coplanar pulses are processed and combined in order to generate a gray scale image. Thus, US transducers act either as a speaker or a microphone. Usually only a small portion of US pulse returns as a reflected echo after reaching a body tissue interface, while most US pulse continues along the beam line to deeper tissues.

B-Mode imaging has a very important clinical impact in patient management as, in real time, it can diagnose CKD, urinary tract obstruction and can indicate treatments and prognosis [2]. Morphological parameters studied with US are kidneys' longitudinal diameter, parenchymal echogenicity and thickness, corticomedullary differentiation, kidneys' profiles, hyperechoic central complex and urinary tract status (fig. 1). Longitudinal diameter is measured in coronal scans and it correlates with calculated volume and renal function. Other renal diameters (anteroposterior and transverse) are not useful in the diagnostic assessment. Kidneys' size immediately distinguishes AKI from CKD, in which both kidneys are small with an altered structure (fig. 2) [2]. In AKI, infiltrative diseases such as monoclonal gammopathy, lymphoma or amyloidosis (fig. 3) are suspected if kidneys' volume is increased with globular aspect, hyperechoic cortex and rounded/hypoechoic pyramids. These features are not specific and they can be observed also in acute proliferative glomerulonephritis with crescents, in acute tubular necrosis and in acute interstitial nephritis [3]. Kidneys are enlarged also in acute renal vein thrombosis and this feature is a very sensitive and specific parameter (>80%) of acute rejection in transplant patients [4].

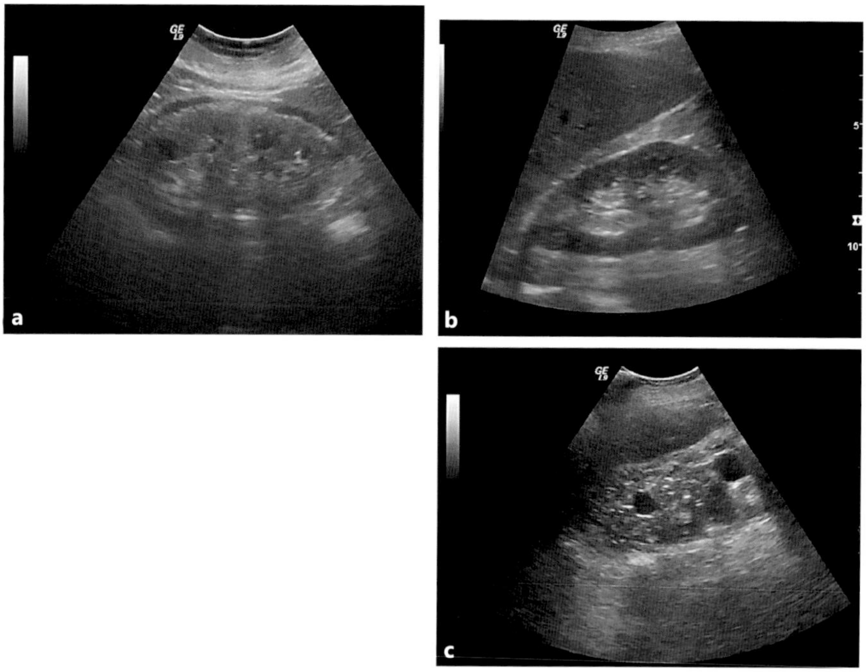

Fig. 2. Morphological features of kidneys in different CKD stages. **a** Drug induced interstitial nephropathy with previous nephrotic syndrome. Kidneys' morphological parameters are: longitudinal diameter 9.3 cm, RI 0.72, serum creatinine (sCr) 2.4 mg/dl, proteinuria 0.7 g/day. **b** severe chronic glomerulonephritis (sCr 3.8 mg/dl; glomerular filtration rate-GFR 23 ml/min). Longitudinal diameter is 7.5 cm with homogeneous parenchyma without cortico-medullary differentiation. **c** Small structureless end-stage kidney, with acquired small cysts, poorly recognizable in the renal lodge.

Renal parenchymal echogenicity is a subjective parameter based on the comparison with liver and spleen echogenicity. Renal cortical and medullary brightness is related to their own different interfaces and structures; so this feature can be influenced by many factors, such as patient habitus, age, hydration, US settings (focus, total gain) and artifacts. From a theoretical point of view, the major determinant of echoes intensity is the structural difference of acoustic impedance between adjacent tissues. In normal kidneys, for example, there is a difference between cortex and medulla acoustic impedance, mainly due to the spatial arrangement of renal tubules. There is also an important difference in impedance between the parenchyma and the fat that surrounds renal sinus structures; so in normal kidneys, it is possible to distinguish the cortex from the medulla and the renal sinus, being the latter highly hyperechoic. Another factor that determines the reflected signal intensity is the tissue density related to the number of reflectors per unit of tissue volume. For example,

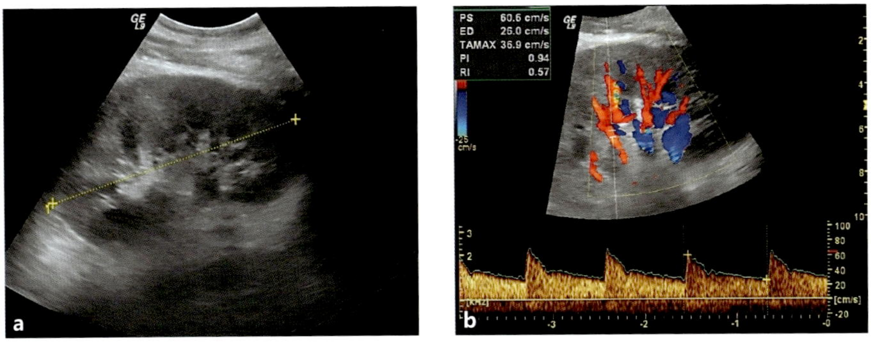

Fig. 3. Membranous glomerulonephritis in lymphoblastic lymphoma treated with bone marrow transplantation. Nephrotic proteinuria and reduced glomerular filtration rate occured after reduction of immunosuppression. **a** Renal morphological findings are non-specific: kidneys' volume is increased with globular aspect, hyperechoic cortex and rounded/hypoechoic pyramids. **b** Intraparenchymal RI 0.57.

renal tissue becomes hypoechoic because of interstitial edema, while it becomes hyperechoic when inflammatory cells infiltrate the interstitium. Examples of hyperechoic kidney are nephropathy during monoclonal gammopathies or multiple myeloma, toxic acute interstitial nephropathy [2], acute proliferative diffuse glomerulonephritis, rapidly progressive glomerulonephritis with crescents and acute pyelonephritis [3]. Cortical thickness can be measured only if medullary pyramids are distinguishable from cortex. In normal adults, cortical thickness is >1 cm above the basal profile of pyramids. Cortical thickness measurement shows a great intra- and inter-operator variability; so it is not a very reliable parameter in the differential diagnosis. In kidneys' morphological evaluation, it is important to determine the corticomedullary thickness near the mesorenal column (fig. 4); this parameter is more reliable than cortex thickness. Parenchymal thickness is a very important parameter that differentiates AKI from CKD. In fact, parenchymal thickness progressively decreases in CKD, showing either a regular profile (glomerular diseases, secondary CKD and interstitial diseases) or an irregular feature (pyelonephritis, obstructive uropathy). Cortical edema and/or infiltration may be suggested by increased cortical thickness, associated with renal globular feature and diffuse hypoechoic pyramids. Increased kidneys' volume is associated with increased thickness and cortical echogenicity in acute tubular necrosis, glomerulonephritis and in acute interstitial nephritis (fig. 5) [2]. However, this parameter shows a high variability; so its use is limited in the absence of a baseline patient evaluation. A hypoechoic perirenal fluid collection is often present in acute cortical necrosis and should not be confused with the hypoechoic perirenal fat present in some patients with CKD.

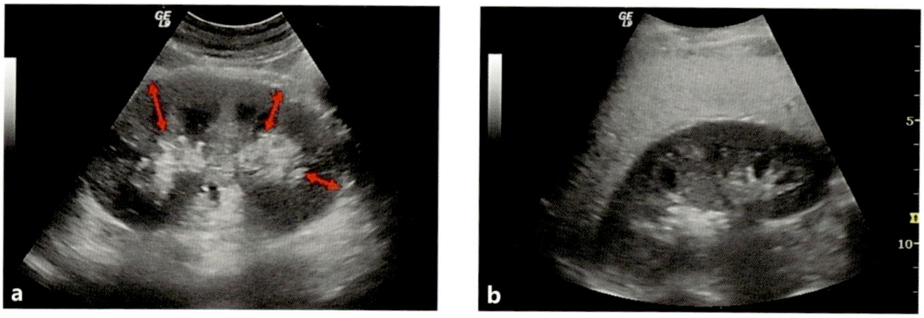

Fig. 4. Cortico-medullary thickness measurement and evaluation of echogenicity. **a** From a morphological point of view, cortico-medullary thickness measurement is a more reliable parameter than cortical parenchymal thickness. **b** Kidneys' echogenicity may vary depending on patient habitus, age, hydration, instrumental parameters (focus, total gain) and artifacts. In this image, renal parenchyma appears hypoechoic due to the attenuation induced by hepatic steatosis.

Conventional US examination is very useful in obstructive post-renal AKI diagnosis (fig. 6). Calyces and pelvis dilation suggests obstruction, but this feature may be evident even in para-physiological conditions as pregnancy or medical conditions that enhance diuresis such as diabetes insipidus. In renal transplant, US sensitivity in the diagnosis of urinary tract obstruction is very high (>90%) [5], while specificity is high only in severe hydronephrosis [2].

Doppler US

Doppler technique measures changes in blood flow velocity and provides indirect information on renal blood flow. Parenchymal 'blushing' is a semi-quantitative parameter strongly influenced by Doppler sensitivity and settings (gain, pulse repetition frequency, filter, focus), and it correlates with cortical diastolic flow impairment and resistance indexes (RI) trend [6]. RIs are recorded on the spectral curve of interlobar arteries, and they provide semi-quantitative information on microcirculation general conditions, thus better characterizing parenchymal damage. Unfortunately, RI measurement becomes difficult in critical care patients with severe cardiorespiratory problems. Moreover, in critical care patients, intrarenal vasomotility is completely altered due to primary disease and pharmacological treatments; so RI diagnostic accuracy decreases if compared with biological markers of early kidney injury (NGAL, cystatin C). In a study of 41 subjects with parenchymal renal disease, RIs were compared with histology and they were much higher in acute tubulointerstitial diseases than they were in acute glomerular diseases (0.75 vs. 0.58, $p < 0.01$) [7]. Moreover, average RI values were significantly

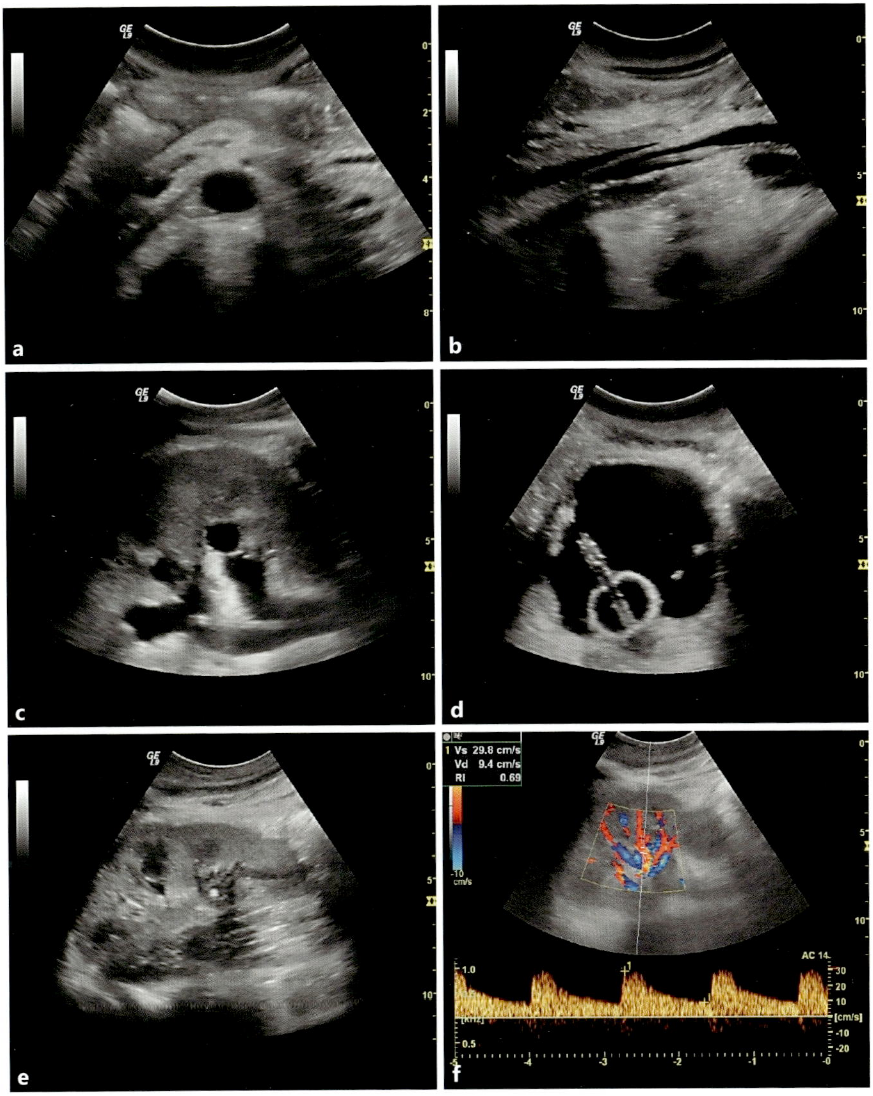

Fig. 5. AKI secondary to drug induced interstitial nephropathy. Male, aged 67. Gastrectomy for gastric cancer and peritoneal carcinomatosis without nodular ascites. **a–c** Double ureteral stent for mesenteric carcinomatosis extended to peri- and pararenal spaces with involvement of renal vessels and ureters. No hydronephrosis with open vesical catheter. Mild hydronephrosis after closing the catheter. **d** AKI (sCr 7 mg/dl) one week after Taxol administration. **e** Right kidney diameter 12.5 cm. Double district and double vascularization. Hyperchoic parenchyma, with well evident and hypoechoic pyramids. Left kidney appears globular, with longitudinal diameter 13 cm and the same structure of the contralateral kidney. **f** Intraparenchymal RI 0.69–0.71.

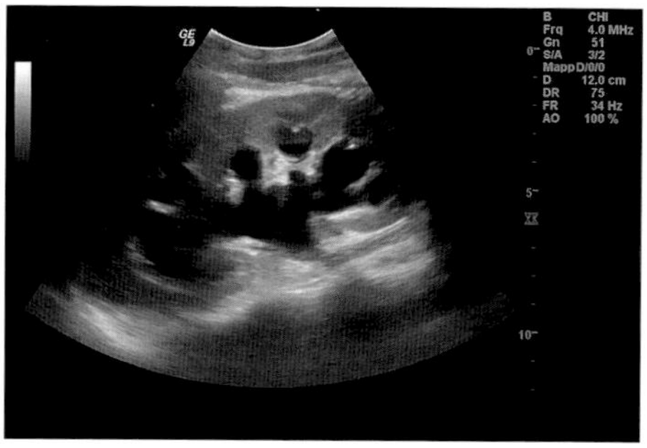

Fig. 6. Hydronephrosis caused by ureteral obstruction. Conventional ultrasonography is the first choice imaging technique in the diagnosis of urinary tract obstruction. In this image, pelvis and calyces are hypoechoic, dilated and rounded.

higher in patients with acute tubular necrosis and vasculitis/degenerative vascular diseases (0.78 and 0.82, respectively) [7]. Typically, RI >0.75 are most commonly associated with acute parenchymal diseases, while RI <0.75 are more common in acute pre-renal diseases. In any case, RI measurement is influenced by Doppler technique and several factors such as age, hypertension and drugs [8].

Contrast-Enhanced Ultrasonography

CEUS is used to evaluate myocardial perfusion in cardiology [9]. US contrast agents are high molecular weight microbubbles of perfluorocarbon or nitrogen gas, with shells of albumin, galactose, lipid or polymers. These contrasts agents are administered intravenously. When microbubbles are reached by an US signal with low mechanical index, they resonate with a specific frequency depending on microbubble diameter, thus generating a second harmonic back signal that reproduces renal macro- and microcirculation. US contrast agents are different from those used in MR and CT because they do not diffuse into the interstitium. Microbubbles diameter (1–6 μm) allows overcoming peripheral and pulmonary capillary bed without hemodynamic effects. Based on these considerations, CEUS should be the perfect imaging technique for the study of renal macro- and microcirculation. But, in practice, perfusion contrastographic imaging provides only qualitative information on microcirculation, and not quantitative information. Dynamic CEUS is the only technique that provides a quantitative evaluation of microcirculation. In this technique, microbubbles reach their maximum dilution in the intrarenal circulation within 2 minutes. At this time, a short sequence of US with high mechanical index (>1) is sent to kidney, and so the microbubbles are destructed. The refilling phase is then analyzed with a low mechanical index (= 0.1); so it is possible to calculate the district flow rate and to compare a region of interest with other renal regions or with the same region in following CEUS evaluations. With dynamic CEUS it is possible to calculate the changes in district flow during the different stages of AKI [10]. In the USA, the FDA has approved CEUS only for blood flow studies on myocardial diseases. The few human studies performed in Europe have shown that dynamic CEUS may be useful in monitoring blood flow in transplantation. There are many parameters that can be analyzed with dynamic CEUS (perfusion velocity, district perfusion); so this method could be used to study blood flow in patients with acute kidney disease, although specific studies are needed to validate this technique. CEUS could be particularly useful in clinical situations in which patient transfer outside the intensive care unit is very difficult.

Conclusion

Grey-scale US is the most common imaging technique used in the first evaluation of patients with AKI or CKD. It is widely available, easy to use and free of complications. Portable US machines represent an important advantage, especially in intensive care units. Basic information provided by B-Mode US about kidney structure includes renal size and cortical echogenicity. Kidney size is a useful parameter in differentiating AKI from CKD. In AKI, an increased kidney volume suggests infiltrative diseases such as lymphoma, monoclonal gammopathies or acute proliferative glomerulonephritis, acute tubular necrosis and acute interstitial nephritis. In kidney transplantation, US features such as increased kidney volume have a sensitivity and specificity greater than 80% in the diagnosis of acute rejection. Cortical thickness not only differentiates AKI from CKD, but may also suggest edema or infiltration of renal cortex. B-Mode US is a very useful imaging modality to exclude urinary tract obstruction as a cause of AKI. Calyceal dilation suggests urinary tract obstruction. US sensitivity in diagnosing urinary tract obstruction in renal allograft is very high (>90%). Color Doppler provides information on renal blood flow. RIs are calculated on the basis of Doppler waveform in main renal artery or smaller intrarenal vessels. Recent advances in US technology allow the study of arteries up to interlobular vessels. In summary, renal US remains the safest, most useful and most widely used imaging technique in the first assessment of patients with AKI. Information on kidney size and echogenicity leads physicians to appropriate decision-making pathways in the management of AKI. CEUS could be a safe and practical tool in the study of renal hemodynamic in the future.

References

1 Platt JF, Ellis JH, Rubin JM, DiPietro MA, Sedman AB: Intrarenal arterial Doppler sonography in patients with nonobstructive renal disease: correlation of resistive index with biopsy findings. AJR Am J Roentgenol 1990;154:1223–1227.

2 O'Neill WC: B-mode sonography in acute renal failure. Nephron Clin Pract 2006; 103:c19–c23.

3 Pozzi Mucelli R, Bertolotto M, Quaia E: Imaging techniques in acute renal failure. Contrib Nephrol 2001;132:76–91.

4 Nicholson ML, Bell A, Burton PR, Donnelly PK, Veitch PS, Bell PR: Probability of rejection predicted from ultrasonographic measurement of renal transplant swelling. Br J Surg 1993;80:1059–1062.

5 Gottlieb RH, Voci SL, Cholewinski SP, Hartley DF, Rubens DJ, Orloff MS, et al: Sonography: a useful tool to detect the mechanical causes of renal transplant dysfunction. J Clin Ultrasound 1999;27:325–333.

6 Turetschek K, Nasel C, Wunderbaldinger P, Diem K, Hittmair K, Mostbeck GH: Power Doppler versus color Doppler imaging in renal allograft evaluation. J Ultrasound Med 1996;15:517–522.

7 Friedrich JO, Adhikari N, Herridge MS, Beyene J: Meta-analysis: low-dose dopamine increases urine output but does not prevent renal dysfunction or death. Ann Intern Med 2005;142:510–524.

8 Quaia E, Bertolotto M: Renal parenchymal diseases: is characterization feasible with ultrasound? Eur Radiol 2002;12:2006–2020.

9 Swinburn JM, Lahiri A, Senior R: Intravenous myocardial contrast echocardiography predicts recovery of dysynergic myocardium early after acute myocardial infarction. J Am Coll Cardiol 2001;38:19–25.

10 Wei K, Le E, Bin JP, Coggins M, Thorpe J, Kaul S: Quantification of renal blood flow with contrast-enhanced ultrasound. J Am Coll Cardiol 2001;37:1135–1140.

Claudio Ronco, MD
Director of Department of Nephrology Dialysis and Transplantation
International Renal Research Institute (IRRIV), San Bortolo Hospital
Viale Rodolfi 37, IT–36100 Vicenza (Italy)
E-Mail cronco@goldnet.it

Meola M, Petrucci I, Ronco C (eds): Ultrasound Imaging in Acute and Chronic Kidney Disease.
Contrib Nephrol. Basel, Karger, 2016, vol 188, pp 21–32 (DOI: 10.1159/000445462)

Clinical Scenarios in Acute Kidney Injury: Pre-Renal Acute Kidney Injury

Mario Meola[a, b] · Federico Nalesso[c] · Ilaria Petrucci[a, b] · Sara Samoni[a, c] · Claudio Ronco[c]

[a]Sant'Anna School of Advanced Studies, Pisa, [b]Department of Internal Medicine, University of Pisa, Pisa, and [c]Department of Nephrology Dialysis and Transplantation, International Renal Research Institute (IRRIV), San Bortolo Hospital, Vicenza, Italy

Abstract

Approximately 70% of community-acquired cases of acute kidney injury are attributed to pre-renal causes. In most of these cases, the underlying kidney function may be normal, but decreased renal perfusion associated with low intravascular volume or decreased arterial pressure can determine a reduced glomerular filtration rate (GFR). Autoregulatory mechanisms can partially compensate renal perfusion reduction in order to maintain GFR. In patients with pre-existing chronic kidney disease, however, these mechanisms are impaired, and the susceptibility to develop acute-on-chronic renal failure is higher.

Introduction

Clinical scenarios of pre-renal acute kidney injury (AKI) are described in some clinical conditions that can be diagnosed by ultrasound (US) and color Doppler (CD). Pre-renal AKI generally recovers within 24–48 h if patient is treated with the appropriate therapy; conversely, initial and functional renal function impairment may evolve into acute tubular necrosis (ATN). Cardiorenal syndrome type 1 and 2 frequently cause AKI (fig. 1). The term 'cardiorenal syndrome' is more and more often used to describe the complex cross-talk between an acute or chronic disease of heart and kidney (cardio-renal syndrome type 1 and 2, respectively) and, vice versa, between an acute or chronic renal dysfunction associated to cardiac dysfunction (cardiorenal syndrome type 3 and 4, respectively). US may be useful in cardiorenal syndrome type 1 (acute renal dysfunction due

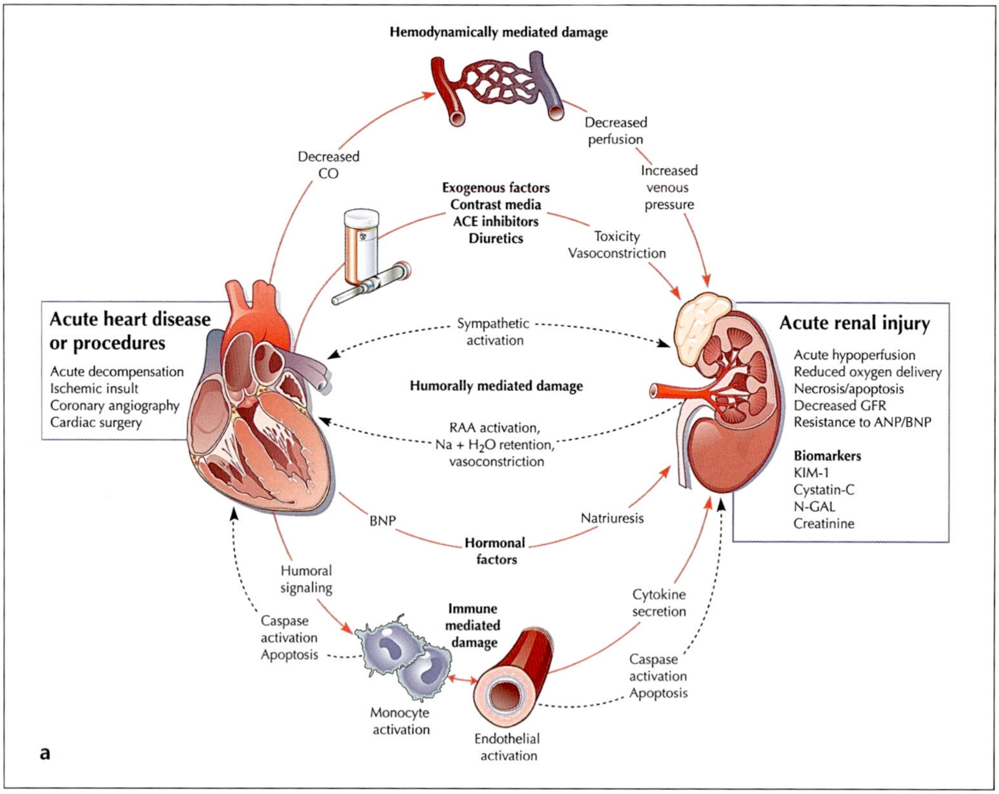

Fig. 1. Cardiorenal syndrome type 1 and 2. **a** Cross-talk between heart and kidney in cardiorenal syndrome type 1 due to acute heart failure (cardiogenic shock, acute heart failure, left/right or biventricular failure). ACE = Angiotensin-converting enzyme; ANP = atrial natriuretic peptide; BNP = B-type natriuretic peptide; GFR = glomerular filtration rate; KIM = kidney injury molecule; N-GAL = neutrophil gelatinase-associated lipocalin; RAA = renin angiotensin aldosterone. LVH = left ventricular hypertrophy. Modified from [1].

to acute heart failure or cardiogenic shock associated with heart failure) and in cardiorenal syndrome type 2 or chronic renal dysfunction related to chronic congestive heart failure [1].

AKI and Left-Ventricle Heart Failure

Heart failure can involve the left and/or right ventricle. Generally, heart failure originates from left ventricle. The signs and symptoms of heart failure vary depending on the cardiac area involved and on disease severity and phase.

Acute left ventricular failure (ischemia, left ventricular hypertrophy) causes a severe fall in the stroke volume, which results in pulmonary congestion, tachy-

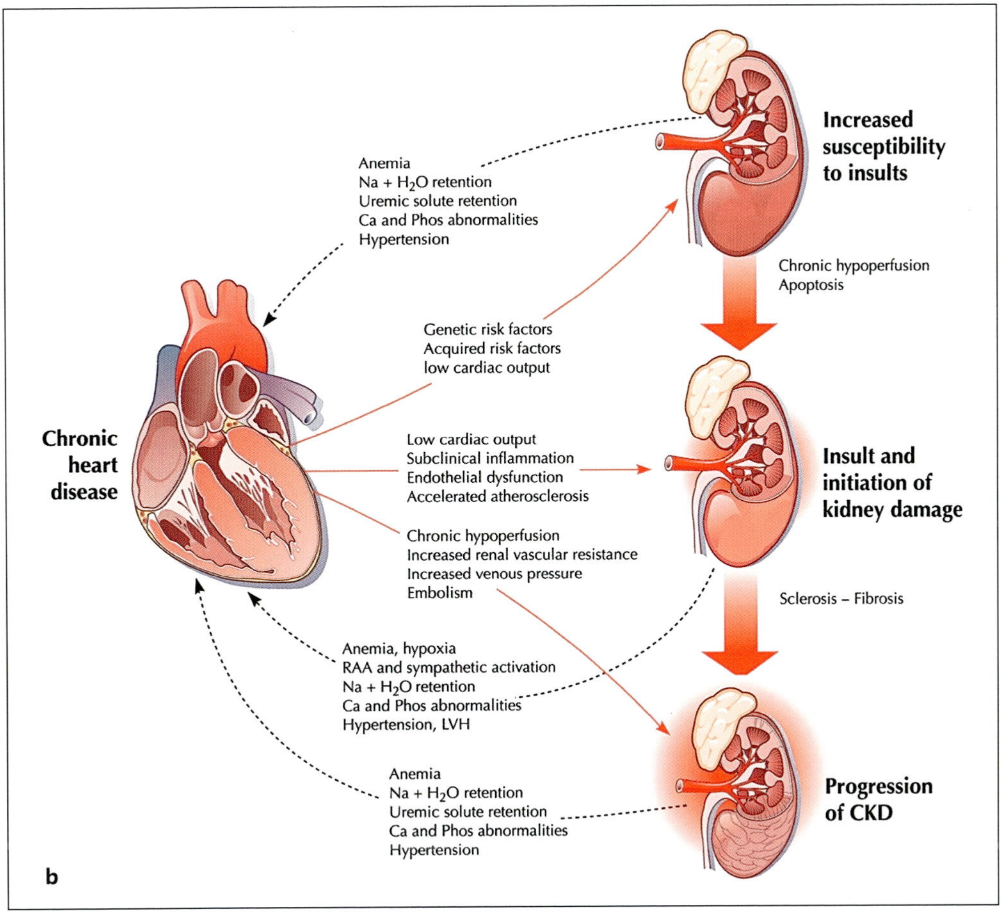

Fig. 1. Cardiorenal syndrome type 1 and 2. **b** Cross-talk between heart and kidney in cardiorenal syndrome type 2 due to chronic congestive heart failure. ACE = Angiotensin-converting enzyme; ANP = atrial natriuretic peptide; BNP = B-type natriuretic peptide; GFR = glomerular filtration rate; KIM = kidney injury molecule; N-GAL = neutrophil gelatinase-associated lipocalin; RAA = renin angiotensin aldosterone. LVH = left ventricular hypertrophy. Modified from [1].

cardia, dyspnea, orthopnea and pulmonary edema. The sudden drop in the ejection fraction leads to visceral organs perfusion impairment with a subsequent peripheral vasoconstriction and blood flow redistribution. Kidneys reduced perfusion, leading to renin-angiotensin-aldosterone system activation, which results in sodium and water retention. These adaptive mechanisms have a different pathophysiologic pathway, depending on acute or chronic features of heart failure. Acute distension of left atrium causes sodium-free diuresis, while chronic distension determines water and sodium retention. Acute right ventricular

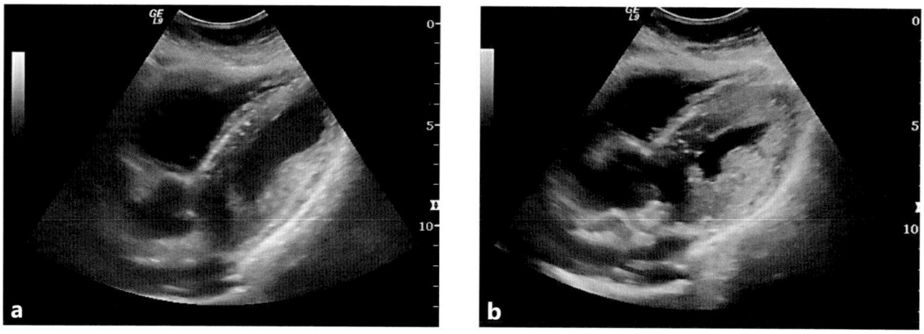

Fig. 2. Subcostal 4-chamber view. Left ventricle hypertrophy (**a**, **b**).

failure (pulmonary hypertension, atrial septal defect, biventricular failure secondary to left ventricular failure, tricuspid valve disease, etc.) leads to systemic venous hypertension with its signs: cyanosis, distended jugular veins, inferior vena cava and hepatic veins congestion, liver and spleen congestion, peripheral edema, pleural and pericardial effusion until anasarcatic state. Oliguria may occur in right or left heart failure, but it is more common in biventricular failure. In this condition, urine osmolality is high (specific gravity ranges from 1,020 to 1,030) while sodium excretion is <20 mEq/l.

In pre-renal AKI, during left ventricular failure, conventional kidney US does not show specific signs. In the absence of pre-existing renal diseases, kidney shows normal volume and parenchymal thickness. Corticomedullary pattern may be normal or diffusely hyperechoic if hypoperfusion is persistent. There are no signs of urinary stasis and bladder is almost empty. Intrarenal resistances are initially low for compensatory pre-glomerular vasodilation, and then they rapidly increase if ischemia is not corrected and functional kidney damage progresses toward ATN. Therefore, the increased differential pressure and the diastolic flow impairment lead to inadequate and pulse parenchymal perfusion. Inferior vena cava appears collapsed, and hepatic veins are not easily detectable. In AKI, secondary to acute decompensate left ventricular failure, the subcostal 4-chamber view may show left ventricle concentric hypertrophy (symmetric or asymmetric; fig. 2) or changes in heart volume associated with more or less extensive ventricular hypokinesia.

Lung Comet Tails

In recent years, chest US has been proposed as the first-line survey to assess the effects of pulmonary congestion on interlobular structures (fig. 3).

In conventional chest radiography, pulmonary capillary congestion and interlobular septal thickening determine the occurrence of Kerley B striae. They

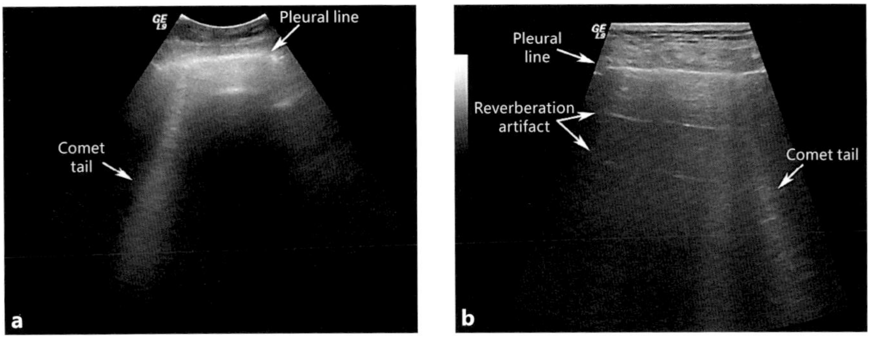

Fig. 3. Comet-tail artifact. This reverberation artifact corresponds to Kerley B striae and it is generated by the intense US beam reflection in hyperhydrated subpleural septa (**a**, **b**).

are thin hyperdense lines, which run near the lung surface. Kerley B striae are commonly <1 cm long, parallel to each other and perpendicular to the pleura, as they represent thickened subpleural interlobular septa. Kerley B striae are usually detectable in peripheral lung areas and bases, while they are missed along pulmonary fissures [2].

In normal conditions, the pleura is the only thoracic anatomical structure visible on conventional US. In intercostal scans, it appears as a thin continuous hyperechoic line, which moves synchronously with breathing. Since pleura in the air-filled lungs is responsible of a specular reflection of US wave, it generates an artifact due to reverberation. Thin hyperechoic lines parallel to each other from the surface to the depth characterize it.

When the lung air content decreases, such as in pulmonary edema or fibrosis, some reflective interfaces appear in subpleural septa (fibrosis/air or air/water). It means that, in pulmonary fibrosis as well as in acute pulmonary edema, US wave crosses subpleural septa, which are thickened by fibrosis or water. The strong reflection of the US wave that occurs at this level creates a reverberation artifact known as 'comet-tail artifact' (fig. 4). This is similar to 'ring-down artifact', that occurs in the stomach when air is mixed with ingested and secretions. In conventional US, the lung comet-tail artifact appears as a thin hyperechoic vertical line that goes, gradually attenuating, from the pleura to the depth. The comet-tail artifact has a continuous vertical movement, synchronous with the breath and similar to a laser beam. The number of lines increases with lung consolidation and the decrease of its air content. When the lung collapses, pleural space is occupied by fluid (transudate or exudate) and atelectatic lung becomes similar to a parenchymal organ, such as the liver and the spleen.

The presence of lung comet-tails can be detected by any US equipment and by any probe (linear, convex, microconvex or sectorial). US examination can

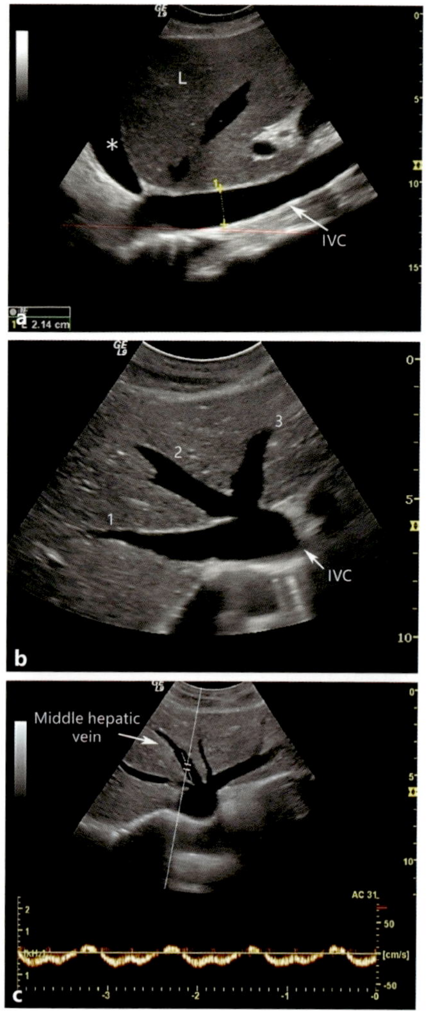

Fig. 4. Right overload. **a** When venous return exceeds the right heart capacity, central venous pressure increases and vena cava appears dilated (anteroposterior diameter >2 cm) and not collapsing. **b** The confluence of hepatic veins appears dilated and hepatic congestion determines hepatomegaly. **c** In systemic congestion, hepatic veins are dilated. The middle hepatic vein is the most suitable sampling site for suprahepatic venogram. L = Liver; IVC = inferior vena cava; * = pleural effusion; 1, 2, 3 = hepatic veins.

also be performed at the bedside. The objective of US examination is to count comet-tails in right and left lung fields of anterior hemithorax. Several methods to standardize US lung examination have been proposed. Right and left hemithorax are commonly studied from the second to the fourth intercostal space (and up to the fifth space on the right side). The assessment of lung comet-tails should be performed along the parasternal, midclavicular, anterior-axillary and medio-axillary lines [3]. The sum of lines measured in each of these spaces creates a score that can be considered a semi-quantitative parameter to evaluate the severity of pulmonary edema. In each space, lines should be numbered from 0 to 10: 0 means no line, while 10 is assigned when US image is completely hyperechoic due to the confluence of lines. In these conditions, to obtain a semi-quantitative parameter, the scan area should be divided by 10 and the percentage of hyperechoic parts should be taken into account [4]. Since lines tend to dissolve in a few minutes after the administration of loop diuretics or after a dialysis treatment with ultrafiltration, the assessment of lung comet-tails may be used for a real-time evaluation of patients' response. Dynamic nature of this artifact has been confirmed by studies in hemodialysis patients, in which the number of lung comet-tails significantly decreased after the correction of dry weight [5].

AKI and Right Heart Failure

Right heart failure is often a complication of left ventricular insufficiency. The pathway by which hemodynamic left failure causes right ventricular impairment is not yet completely clear. Biventricular failure and increased filling pressures cause pulmonary and systemic venous hypertension, thus determining congestive heart failure. Conventional US and CD are very useful in the diagnosis of AKI associated with right heart failure and congestive heart failure (low output syndrome). In the subcostal 4-chamber view, the morphology of the 4 heart chambers may show cardiomegaly, diffuse hypokinesis, right atrium dilation and, in cases of bi-ventricular heart failure, left ventricle hypertrophy. When venous return exceeds the capacity of the right heart, central venous pressure increases. In this hemodynamic situation, inferior vena cava and hepatic veins are dilated and liver capillary congestion causes an increase in liver volume.

At US, vena cava appears dilated (anteroposterior diameter >2 cm) and rigid, the confluence of suprahepatic veins is dilated and their intrahepatic course is evident (fig. 4). Inferior vena cava diameter does not change during breathing, cardiac cycle and with probe mechanical compression [6]. Inferior vena cava rigidity has led some authors to consider its anteroposterior diameter as a parameter for the identification of fluid overload not only in the diagnosis of right heart failure but also in dialysis patients. After the initial enthusiasm, this measure has been replaced by bioimpendence, because inferior vena cava diameter shows a high intra- and inter-individual variability.

Congestive Hepatopathy

Congestive liver shows homogeneous structure with rounded profiles. Increased volume can be measured with cranio-caudal diameter of the right lobe in a longitudinal scan along the emiclavear line. A diameter >13 cm is indicative of

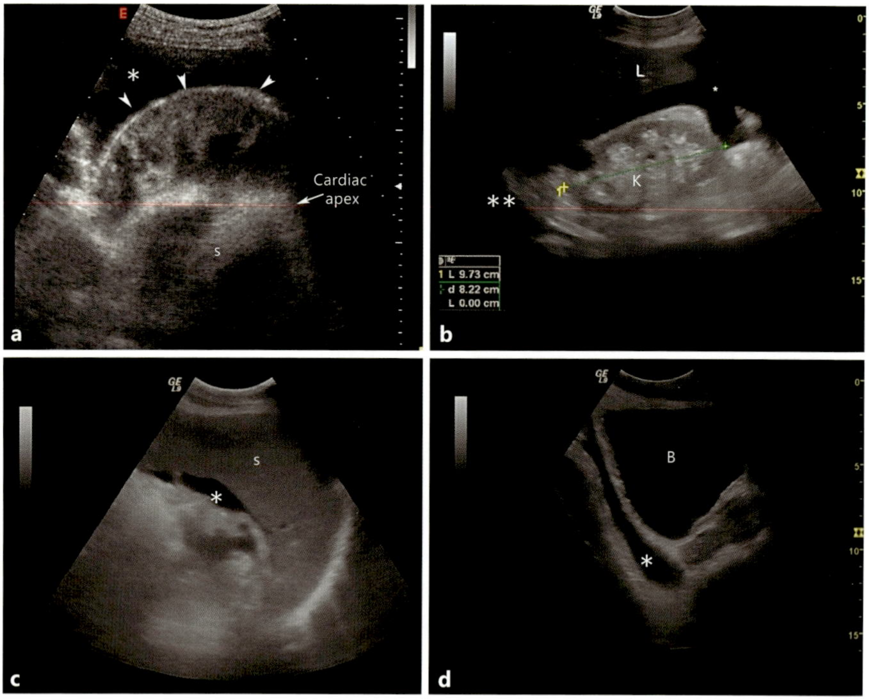

Fig. 5. Pleural, pericardic effusion and ascites in right heart failure. **a** Pleural and pericardic chronic effusion. US shows hyperechoic fibrin bridles. * = Pleural effusion; S = interventricular septum; arrowheads = pericardial flap front. **b** Thin layer of ascites in subhepatic Morrison's space. L = Liver; K = kidney; * = ascites; ** = pleural effusion. **c** Thin effusion in perisplenic space. S = Spleen; * peri-splenic effusion. **d** Thin effusion in the Douglas pouch. B = Bladder; * = ascites.

hepatomegaly. During right heart failure with AKI, a modest right pleural effusion may occur.

If pleural fluid is an exudate, pleural effusion appears anechoic with hyperechoic fibrin septa, which float in the pleural space or fix the lung to the pleura. A thin layer of ascites is present in subhepatic recess (Morrison's pouch) and in the peri-splenic region, a modest effusion can also be present in the pouch of Douglas (fig. 5); a thin pericardial effusion confirms the trend to anasarcatic state. These findings are present either in right heart failure, in nephrotic syndrome with anasarcatic state or in underdialyzed patients with fluid overload. Spleen is usually not increased in volume, although the hilum is congested, while kidneys appear globular, enlarged and diffusely hypoechoic. Renal vein is patent but it may show Doppler modulations similar to those of the inferior vena cava and hepatic veins.

Nevertheless, suprahepatic venogram evaluation is difficult to perform in clinical practice without a real-time ECG, in order to correlate Doppler waves with cardiac activity. Congestion of liver sinusoids causes compression, atrophy and center-lobular necrosis. In the early phases, this congestion determines hepatic steatosis, while in chronic heart failure it causes fibrosis (cirrhosis heart). Perisinusoidal fibrosis, observed in cardiac cirrhosis, reduces parenchymal elasticity, slows venous flow and alters hepatic venogram morphology, which tends to become monophasic. Centripetal speed flow is reduced mainly due to pressure overload of the right atrium. Alternatively, when there is also tricuspid regurgitation, suprahepatic vein pulsatility increases and blood flow during the right systole is reduced or reversed.

Tricuspid Regurgitation

Doppler analysis of S and D waves in the hepatic veins venogram requires some pathophysiologic considerations. In normal venogram, S wave is larger (or equal) than D wave because the systolic tricuspid annulus excursion to the apex facilitates the blood return to the heart. In heart diseases leading to right heart failure with systemic overload, as well as tricuspid insufficiency, right heart is insufficient so it becomes much more evident the diastolic retrograde flow. Severe tricuspid regurgitation is a paradigm to understand the changes in the different stages of regurgitation as in right heart failure [7]. When atrial systole begins, the atrial contraction pushes blood into the ventricle by anterograde flow and retrograde flow to the liver, thus causing the small A wave. During the systole, ventricular contraction stretches the tricuspid annulus toward the cardiac apex. If valvular insufficiency is present, during the rapid filling phase, there is an overlap of blood regurgitation from the ventricle to the right atrium, vena cava and liver caused by tricuspid incontinence. This determines a reduction of S wave amplitude or the appearance of a retrograde S wave. When the ventricle starts to relax and tricuspid annulus returns toward the original position, blood flows back again from the atrium to the vena cava and liver, generating the retrograde V wave. During diastole, tricuspid valve is opened, myocardium is at rest, and blood flows passively from the liver and vena cava to the heart, generating the anterograde D wave, with increased amplitude if compared to normal wave. The degree of tricuspid regurgitation influences the morphology of the suprahepatic venogram, which is classified in grade 1, 2 and 3 (M or W morphology). Grade 1 regurgitation reflects a low reflux, while grade 2 and 3 relate with a mild and severe regurgitation. Hepatic venous flow becomes biphasic when a single retrograde and anterograde wave is identified in each cardiac cycle. This occurs when A, S and V waves are retrograde so a single reverse wave is represented together with an anterograde D wave. This spectral morphology results from right heart failure associated with tricuspid regurgitation.

Right Heart Failure

Venogram morphology of hepatic veins in right heart failure is similar to that in tricuspid regurgitation. Typically, in the early stages of heart failure, there is increased amplitude of retrograde A wave because ventricle during the atrial systole is no longer able to receive all the flow from the right atrium [8]. Since the amplitude of A wave varies, even in normal conditions, this venogram aspect is hardly appreciable. As ventricular failure progresses, reversal relationship between S and D waves becomes more and more evident until S wave reaches the zero line and shows a morphology similar to that of tricuspid regurgitation grade 2 (fig. 6).

This morphology indicates the absence of anterograde flow during ventricular systole.

Constrictive Pericarditis

Doppler analysis of hepatic veins is very important in constrictive pericarditis. The first signs of this pericarditis may be liver stasis or liver disease with increased transaminases, hepatomegaly and ascites [9]. In serum-fibrinous pericarditis, conventional US can show the signs of right overload and the presence of pleural and pericardial effusion with fibrin bridles (fig. 7). Doppler analysis in constrictive pericarditis shows a triphase waveform with a retrograde extra wave at the end of diastole between D and A waves. Since right atrium and ventricle are passively filled through superior and inferior vena cava during diastole (D-wave), right heart capacitance is prematurely reached because of reactive pericardial effusion that determines cardiac constriction. This leads to a retrograde wave to the liver at the end of diastole (fig. 7). The additional reverse wave becomes more prominent during expiration [9, 10].

In severe right heart failure, as in those hemodynamic conditions that reduce right ventricular filling (constrictive pericarditis, restrictive cardiomyopathy, pericardial effusion), venous pulse amplitude increases during inspiration. On the contrary, in normal conditions, venous pulse amplitude decreases during inspiration. This paradox is known as Kussmaul sign.

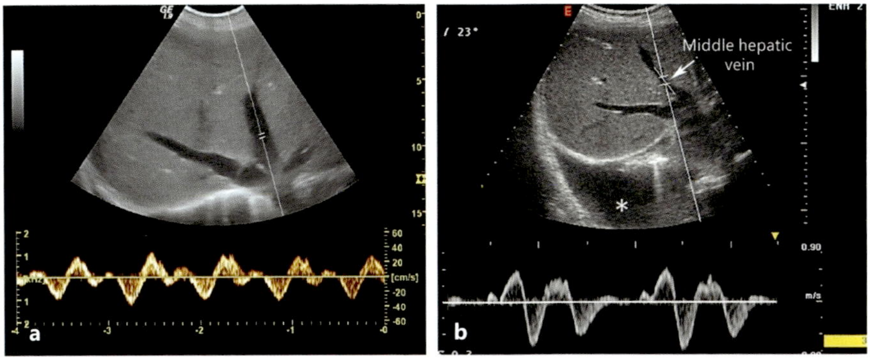

Fig. 6. Venogram in right heart failure with tricuspid regurgitation. **a–c** As ventricular failure worsens, the inversion of ratio between S and D waves appears until S wave reaches the zero line. The differential diagnosis of a biphasic venogram due to tricuspid regurgitation or to right heart failure associated with tricuspid regurgitation is very difficult without an echocardiographic diagnosis and a simultaneous ECG. * = Pleural effusion.

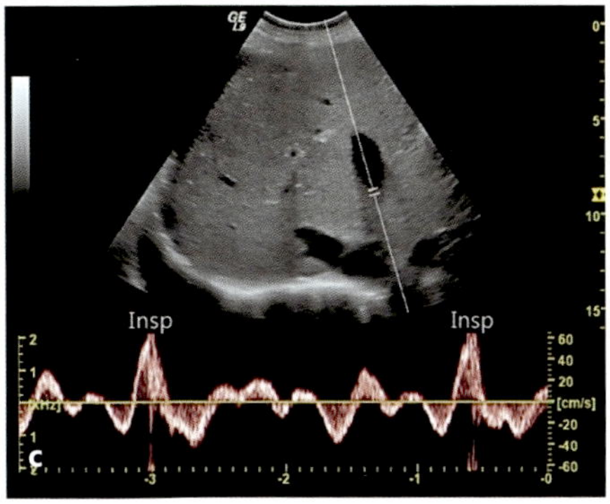

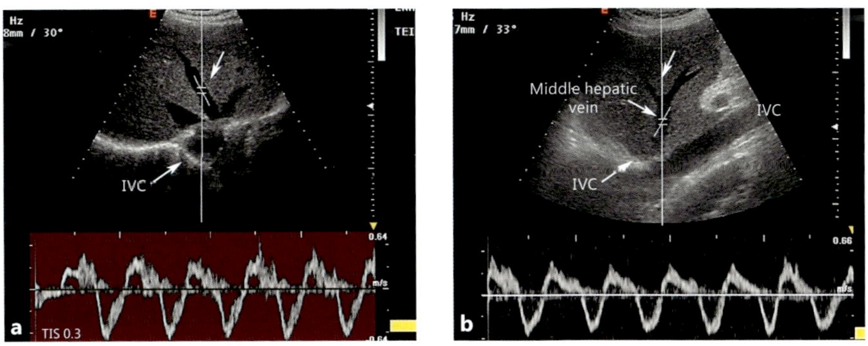

Fig. 7. Venogram morphological patterns during pericarditis with severe effusion. (**a**) Transversal and (**b**) parasagittal scan on inferior vena cava. Cardiac filling is hindered because of severe effusion, so a biphasic wave appears together with a retrograde wave to the liver at the end of diastole. This wave becomes more prominent during the expiratory phase. IVC = Inferior vena cava; white arrow = middle hepatic vein.

Conclusion

B-Mode analysis of the 4 cardiac chambers and pericardium cavity provides important information about cardiac function and regional kinetic of ventricles. Doppler analysis of the vena cava and suprahepatic veins also provides important information about systemic congestion and right atrium pressure. All these parameters are essential in order to evaluate renal hemodynamics and its alterations in cardiorenal syndrome type 1 and 2.

The analysis of comet-tails and the diameter/collapsibility of vena cava also provide information about patient's hydration status and can be use as a parameter for the management of therapy.

References

1 Ronco C, Haapio M, House AA, Anavekar N, Bellomo R: Cardiorenal syndrome. J Am Coll Cardiol 2008;52:1527–1539.

2 Padley SP, Hansell DM, Flower CD, Jennings P: Comparative accuracy of high resolution computed tomography and chest radiography in the diagnosis of chronic diffuse infiltrative lung disease. Clin Radiol 1991;44:222–226.

3 Picano E, Frassi F, Agricola E, Gligorova S, Gargani L, Mottola G: Ultrasound lung comets: a clinically useful sign of extravascular lung water. J Am Soc Echocardiogr 2006;19:356–363.

4 Agricola E, Bove T, Oppizzi M, Marino G, Zangrillo A, Margonato A, Picano E: 'Ultrasound comet-tail images': a marker of pulmonary edema: a comparative study with wedge pressure and extravascular lung water. Chest 2005;127:1690–1695.

5 Mallamaci F, Benedetto FA, Tripepi R, Rastelli S, Castellino P, Tripepi G, Picano E, Zoccali C: Detection of pulmonary congestion by chest ultrasound in dialysis patients. JACC Cardiovasc Imaging 2010;3:586–594.

6 Mandelbaum A, Ritz E: Vena cava diameter measurement for estimation of dry weight in haemodialysis patients. Nephrol Dial Transplant 1996;11(suppl 2):24–27.

7 Abu-Yousef MM: Duplex Doppler sonography of the hepatic vein in tricuspid regurgitation. AJR Am J Roentgenol 1991;156:79–83.

8 Allan PL, Dubbins PA, Poznik MA, McDicken WN: Clinical Doppler Ultrasound. London, Churchill Livingstone, 2000, pp 147–148.

9 Gorka TS, Gorka W: Doppler sonographic diagnosis of severe portal vein pulsatility in constrictive pericarditis: flow normalization after pericardiectomy. J Clin Ultrasound 1999;27:84–88.

10 Von Bibra H, Schober K, Jenni R, Busch R, Sebening H, Blömer H: Diagnosis of constrictive pericarditis by pulsed Doppler echocardiography of the hepatic vein. Am J Cardiol 1989;63:483–488.

Claudio Ronco, MD
Director of Department of Nephrology Dialysis and Transplantation
International Renal Research Institute (IRRIV), San Bortolo Hospital
Viale Rodolfi 37, IT–36100 Vicenza (Italy)
E-Mail cronco@goldnet.it

Meola M, Petrucci I, Ronco C (eds): Ultrasound Imaging in Acute and Chronic Kidney Disease.
Contrib Nephrol. Basel, Karger, 2016, vol 188, pp 33–38 (DOI: 10.1159/000445465)

Clinical Scenarios in Acute Kidney Injury: Hepatorenal Syndrome

Mario Meola[a, b] · Federico Nalesso[c] · Ilaria Petrucci[a, b] · Sara Samoni[a, c] · Claudio Ronco[c]

[a]Sant'Anna School of Advanced Studies, Pisa, [b]Department of Internal Medicine, University of Pisa, Pisa, and [c]Department of Nephrology Dialysis and Transplantation, International Renal Research Institute (IRRIV), San Bortolo Hospital, Vicenza, Italy

Abstract

Renal failure commonly occurs in patients affected by cirrhosis, especially when there is ascites. It is typically secondary to intercurrent events that can further compromise blood flow in conditions of relatively decreased renal perfusion. Hepatorenal syndrome (HRS) is a particular and common type of kidney failure that affects patients with liver cirrhosis or, less frequently, with fulminant hepatic failure. The syndrome is characterized by splanchnic vasodilation and renal vasoconstriction. The classification of HRS identifies 2 categories of kidney failure, known as type 1 and type 2 HRS, that occur in patients with either cirrhosis or fulminant hepatic failure.

Hepatorenal Syndrome

The hepatorenal syndrome (HRS) is one of the most common causes of acute kidney injury (AKI) in patients with acute or chronic liver diseases. Its annual incidence in patients with ascites is about 8% [1]. Affected patients usually not only have portal hypertension due to cirrhosis, severe alcoholic hepatitis or (less often) metastatic tumors but can also have fulminant hepatic failure from any cause [2]. The HRS represents the end stage of a progressive decrease in renal perfusion due to the worsening of hepatic injury. The HRS is a diagnosis of exclusion and it is associated with a poor prognosis [3].

In patients with cirrhosis, AKI may be triggered by hypovolemia (gastrointestinal bleeding, fluid loss, sepsis) or by acute tubular necrosis related to drug administration (non-steroidal anti-inflammatory drugs, aminoglycosides, contrast media). The overlap between AKI and cirrhosis has a negative prognostic significance, and it is an independent predictor of death. Actually, patients with cirrhosis and ascites have a latent functional AKI due to arterial hypotension, hypovolemic status and decreased renal blood flow [4]. This may result in a reduction in glomerular filtration rate (GFR), according to the response of intrarenal autoregulation mechanisms. On the contrary, the onset of complications, the administration of drugs or the use of contrast media may precipitate the situation leading to an acute tubular necrosis.

In advanced liver diseases, AKI can also develop with a specific syndrome known as HRS. It is a type of prerenal AKI that occurs acutely (type 1) or chronically (type 2) in patients with normal renal function and without kidney abnormalities. For this reason, HRS is defined as a pre-renal AKI, despite its frequent irreversibility [5].

The main pathophysiological characteristic of HRS is the extreme renal vasoconstriction associated with the peripheral arteriolar vasodilation. Tubular function is maintained and both proteinuria and kidney histological damage are missed. Authors have identified 2 subtypes of HRS: HRS type 1 is a rapidly progressive renal failure (fig. 1) characterized by a doubling of serum creatinine (sCr) values up to ≥2.5 mg/dl or by a 50% reduction of creatinine clearance until values <20 ml/min, within 2 weeks. On the contrary, HRS type 2 is a moderate renal failure, characterized by sCr >1.5 mg/dl, chronically. While in HRS type 1 the cause is commonly identified, in HRS type 2 AKI is due to refractory ascites [5].

In HRS, renal failure is triggered by a marked vasoconstriction that occurs with not well identified mechanisms [6]. In fact, at the time of diagnosis of HRS, the rapid increase of sCr is not accompanied by shock, loss of fluids, nephrotoxic drugs administration, gastrointestinal bleeding or sepsis. Moreover, renal failure does not improve with plasma expanders or diuretics withdrawal.

Patients with HRS have very high values of renal resistive indexes (RIs; 0.79 ± 0.6; fig. 2). Platt et al. [7] measured RI in 180 patients with chronic liver disease and without renal insufficiency. They demonstrated that RIs are an independent predictor of renal dysfunction and HRS. In patients with early cirrhosis (Child-Pugh A), RI was 0.6 ± 0.07; in patients with cirrhosis B, RI was 0.72 ± 0.08; while

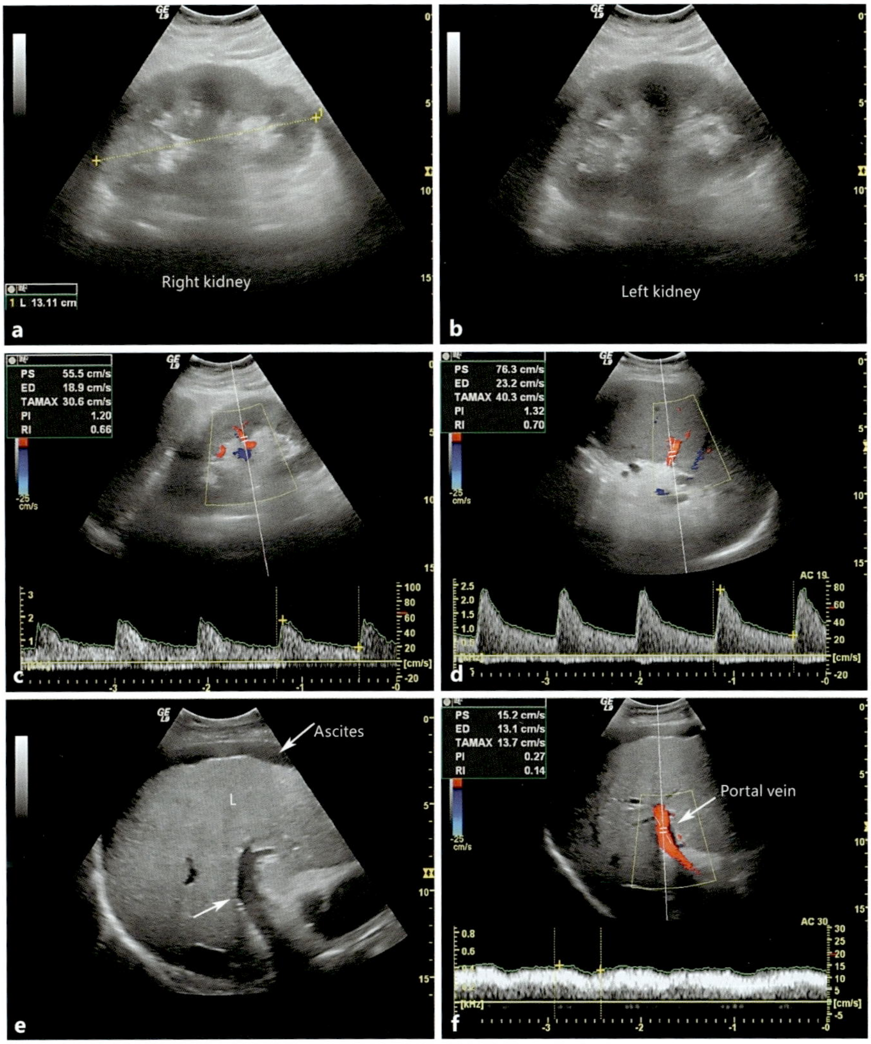

Fig. 1. HRS. Male, aged 57 years, with HCV-related chronic hepatitis from the age of 30 years, with normal renal function. After infectious episode of the upper respiratory and cephalosporin therapy, patient develops AKI (sCr 8.6 mg/dl, AST147 IU/l, ALT 108 IU/l, γGT 118 IU/l, albumin 3.1 g/dl). After the antibiotic stop, without hydration or diuretics, in 24 h, sCr reaches values of 5.4 mg/dl. **a**, **b** Kidneys increased in volume (about 12.5 cm), globular morphology, with widespread structural hypoechogenicity and reduced parenchymal corticomedullary differentiation. **c** Intrarenal RI = 0.66. **d** Splenomegaly with longitudinal dimater >15 cm and intraparenchymal RI 0.70. **e** Mild effusion ascites. Liver with irregular profiles and macronodular degeneration. White arrow = portal vein. **f** Portal vein flow. Splenomegaly and ascites indicates a mild portal hypertension. L = Liver.

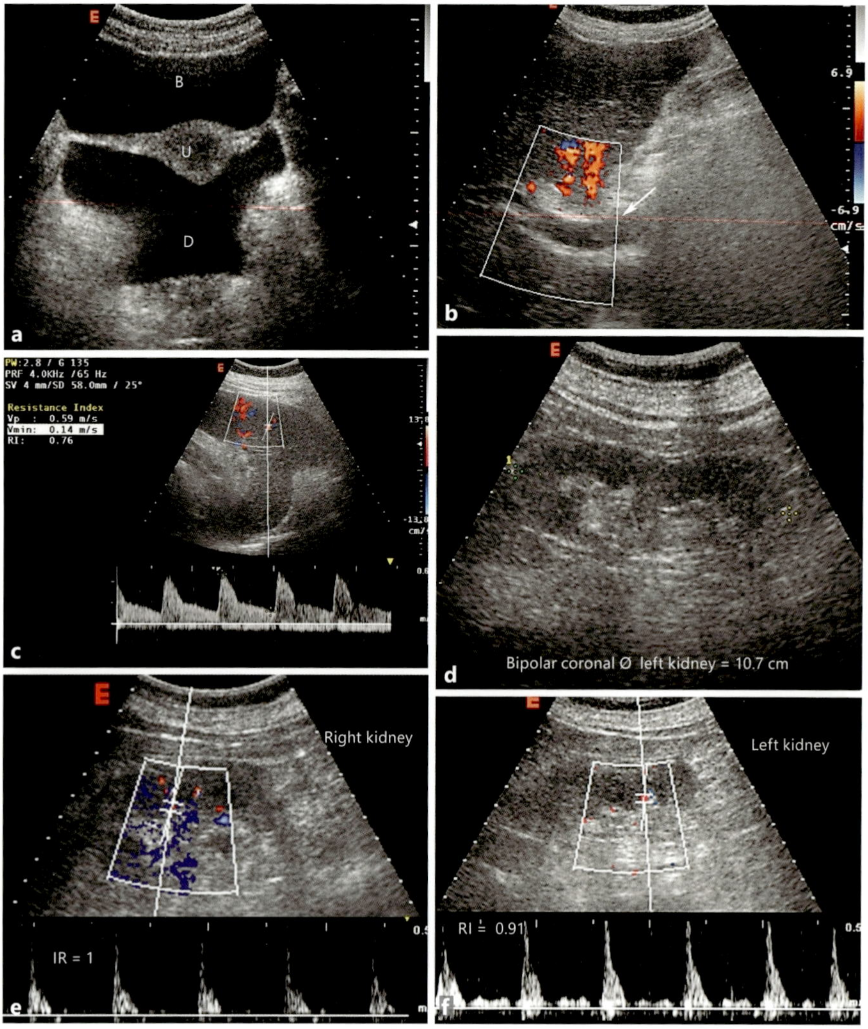

Fig. 2. HRS. Cirrhosis is a predisposing condition to AKI. In patients with ascites and with normal renal function, the intrarenal RIs are higher at baseline than in patients without ascites (0.70 vs. 0.61). HRS is a pre-renal failure that acutely occurs in cirrhotic patients with preserved renal function due to vasoconstriction favored by mechanisms yet unknown. In this case, the patient showed ascites in the pelvic cavity (**a**), portal vein thrombosis (**b**) and moderate splenomegaly (**c**) with vascular congestion (intrasplenic RI 0.76). Both kidneys showed a morphology compatible with age (**d**), but at color Doppler renal perfusion is almost absent. **e**, **f** Intraparenchymal RIs were not easy to sample due to low flow and they were >0.90. Patient died. B = Bladder; U = uterus; D = Douglas pouch with pelvic effusion; Ø = diameter.

in patients with cirrhosis C, RI was 0.74 ± 0.06. Moreover, RIs were significantly different in cirrhotic patients with or without ascites (0.70 ± 0.04 vs. 0.61 ± 0.05). Therefore, serial measurements of RI in patients with liver disease may select a subset of patients without kidney failure but at high risk for AKI and HRS [7]. The increase in RI precedes the increase of sCr and it is an index of reduced survival [8].

Conclusion

The HRS is a frequent complication in patients with cirrhosis, ascites and advanced liver failure. It is a functional renal failure due to renal vasoconstriction and low renal perfusion [3]. Kidney histology is normal or can show lesions, which do not justify the decrease in GFR. Nevertheless, during the last decade, several features suggested a much more complex pathogenesis than the traditional 'peripheral arterial vasodilation hypothesis', which linked HRS to the extreme renal vasoconstriction associated with the splanchnic vasodilation. According to this point of view, 2 types of HRS with different clinical course, prognostic implications and treatment response have been identified. The HRS type 1 and type 2 are not different expressions of a common disorder, but probably 2 different syndromes with a well distinct pathogenesis. The HRS type 1 is an extremely unstable condition. It develops in the setting of acute clinical events, which act as precipitating factors leading to a rapid deterioration of circulatory and renal function, with severe arterial hypotension and acute renal failure with oliguria. This clinical scenario is accompanied by a rapid deterioration of hepatic function, with increase in jaundice and encephalopathy [9]. On the contrary, HRS type 2 is chronic and it develops gradually in patients with cirrhosis and ascites (in stable clinical conditions) and responds poorly to diuretics. Renal vascularization and function remains stable during months or progress slowly, until HRS type 2 occurs.

References

1 Ginès A, Escorsell A, Ginès P, et al: Incidence, predictive factors, and prognosis of the hepatorenal syndrome in cirrhosis with ascites. Gastroenterology 1993;105:229–236.

2 Ginès P, Schrier RW: Renal failure in cirrhosis. N Engl J Med 2009;361:1279–1290.

3 Ginès P, Guevara M, Arroyo V, Rodés J: Hepatorenal syndrome. Lancet 2003;362:1819–1827.

4 Moreau R, Lebrec D: Acute renal failure in patients with cirrhosis: perspectives in the age of MELD. Hepatology 2003;37:233–243.

5 Moore K: The hepatorenal syndrome. Clin Sci (Lond) 1997;92:433–443.
6 Wong F, Blendis L: New challenge of hepatorenal syndrome: prevention and treatment. Hepatology 2001;34:1242–1251.
7 Platt JF, Ellis JH, Rubin JM, Merion RM, Lucey MR: Renal duplex Doppler ultrasonography: a noninvasive predictor of kidney dysfunction and hepatorenal failure in liver disease. Hepatology 1994;20:362–369.
8 Maroto A, Ginès A, Saló J, Clària J, Ginès P, Anibarro L, Jiménez W, Arroyo V, Rodés J: Diagnosis of functional kidney failure of cirrhosis with Doppler sonography: prognostic value of resistive index. Hepatology 1994; 20(4 pt 1):839–844.
9 Sherman DS, Fish DN, Teitelbaum I: Assessing renal function in cirrhotic patients: problems and pitfalls. Am J Kidney Dis 2003;41: 269–278.

Claudio Ronco, MD
Director of Department of Nephrology Dialysis and Transplantation
International Renal Research Institute (IRRIV), San Bortolo Hospital
Viale Rodolfi 37, IT–36100 Vicenza (Italy)
E-Mail cronco@goldnet.it

Meola M, Petrucci I, Ronco C (eds): Ultrasound Imaging in Acute and Chronic Kidney Disease.
Contrib Nephrol. Basel, Karger, 2016, vol 188, pp 39–47 (DOI: 10.1159/000445466)

Clinical Scenarios in Acute Kidney Injury: Parenchymal Acute Kidney Injury-Tubulo-Interstitial Diseases

Mario Meola[a, b] • Sara Samoni[a, c] • Ilaria Petrucci[a, b] • Claudio Ronco[c]

[a]Sant'Anna School of Advanced Studies, Pisa, [b]Department of Internal Medicine, University of Pisa, Pisa, and [c]Department of Nephrology Dialysis and Transplantation, International Renal Research Institute (IRRIV), San Bortolo Hospital, Vicenza, Italy

Abstract

Acute tubular necrosis (ATN) is the most common type of acute kidney injury (AKI) related to parenchymal damage (90% of cases). It may be due to a direct kidney injury, such as sepsis, drugs, toxins, contrast media, hemoglobinuria and myoglobinuria, or it may be the consequence of a prolonged systemic ischemic injury. Conventional ultrasound (US) shows enlarged kidneys with hypoechoic pyramids. Increased volume is largely sustained by the increase of anteroposterior diameter, while longitudinal axis usually maintains its normal length. Despite the role of color Doppler in AKI still being debated, many studies demonstrate that renal resistive indexes (RIs) vary on the basis of primary disease. Moreover, several studies assessed that higher RI values are predictive of persistent AKI. Nevertheless, due to the marked heterogeneity among the studies, further investigations focused on timing of RI measurement and test performances are needed. Acute interstitial nephritis is also a frequent cause of AKI, mainly due to non-steroidal anti-inflammatory drugs and antibiotics administration. The development of acute interstitial nephritis is due to an immunological reaction against nephritogenic exogenous antigens, processed by tubular cells. In acute interstitial nephritis, as well as in ATN, conventional US does not allow a definitive diagnosis. Kidneys appear enlarged and widely hyperechoic due to interstitial edema and inflammatory infiltration. Also, in this condition, hemodynamic changes are closely correlated to the severity and the progression of the anatomical damage.

Introduction

Tubulointerstitial diseases are the main cause of parenchymal acute kidney injury (AKI). Acute tubular necrosis (ATN), which is responsible for 90% of cases of parenchymal AKI, may be due to ischemic or toxic damage. Toxins involved may be exogenous, such as drugs and contrast media, as well as endogenous, such as myoglobin, and myeloma proteins. Acute interstitial nephritis may be due to allergic, infective or infiltrative processes.

Acute Tubular Necrosis

ATN is the most common type of AKI related to parenchymal damage. It may be due to a direct kidney injury, such as sepsis, drugs, toxins, contrast media, hemoglobinuria and myoglobinuria, or it may be the consequence of a prolonged systemic ischemic injury.

In non-nephropathic patients, kidneys could maintain normal size. However, more frequently, conventional ultrasound (US) shows enlarged and globose-shaped kidneys with marked, rounded and hypoechoic pyramids. Increased volume and diffuse hypoechogenicity of pyramids are related to water retention and interstitial edema. These alterations are only partially correlated to the severity of functional and histological damage. Cortex usually maintains normal echogenicity and, only in few cases (about 10%) [1], it may appear widely hyperechoic. This last pattern is more frequent in ATN due to nephrotoxic agents (fig. 1). However, even in post-surgical AKI, conventional US shows enlarged and swollen kidneys with a hypoechoic medulla and a widely hyperechoic cortex (fig. 2) [2].

Increased volume is largely sustained by the increase of anteroposterior diameter, while the longitudinal axis usually maintains its normal length. Kidneys become globose-shaped with a high increase in anteroposterior/longitudinal diameter ratio (>0.53; normal value: 0.45 ± 0.04). The anteroposterior/longitudinal diameter ratio directly correlates with serum creatinine (sCr) values and with severity of hyperpotassemia. On the contrary, it is inversely correlated with urinary osmolarity, which is an index of tubule integrity [3]. In fact, pre-renal diseases are characterized by urinary osmolarity >500 mOsm/kg H_2O, while parenchymal diseases by values <350 mOsm/kg H_2O.

Severe tubular damage can be due to toxins or drugs assumption as well as several pathologic conditions that secondarily affect tubules, such as rapidly progressive glomerulonephritis, acute interstitial nephritis, lupus nephritis and renal lymphoma. There are no US pathognomonic patterns of ATN that allow discerning different disease etiology. However, color Doppler US can show hemodynamic variation, thus consenting differential diagnosis of different types of AKI [4]. Nevertheless, the role of color Doppler in AKI is still debated. In fact some clinicians still consider US to be useless in the management of critically ill patients who does not have physical sings of obstructive nephropathy [5].

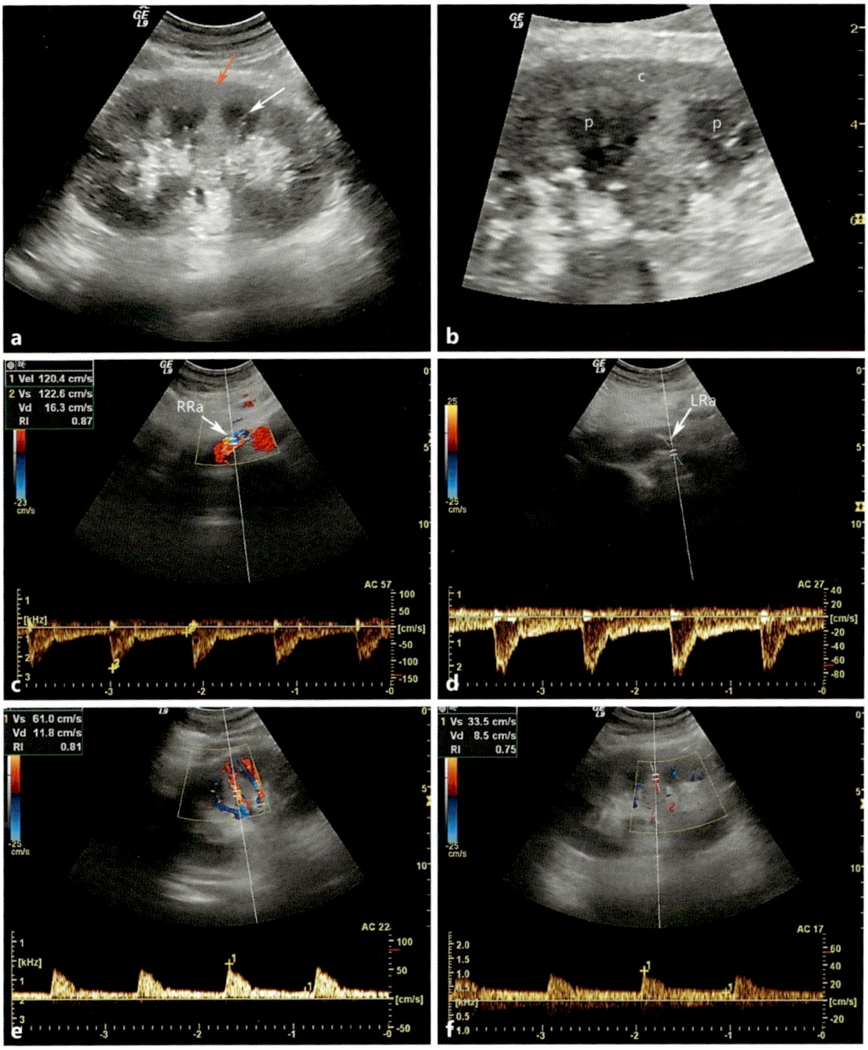

Fig. 1. ATN due to anticryptogamics. Male, aged 39 years. Twelve hours after the abuse of anticryptogamics, he was referred to nephrologist because of oliguria and rapid increase of sCr up to 3.9 mg/dl (**a**, **b**). At B-mode US examination, both kidneys were enlarged (coronal diameter >12.5 cm), globose-shaped with a hyperechoic cortex (red arrow) and irregular and not well distinguished pyramids (white arrow). Color Doppler sampling of right (**c**) and left renal artery (**d**) showed a severe reduction of diastolic velocity due to the increase of intrarenal resistances and flow redistribution. **e**, **f** Parenchymal blushing decreased and perfusion became evident only by using a low pulse repetition frequency. Color Doppler sampling of interlobar arteries showed a diffuse increase of renal RIs from 0.75 to 0.81, revealing a widespread tubular damage. c = Cortex; p = medullary pyramids; RRa = right renal artery; LRa = left renal artery.

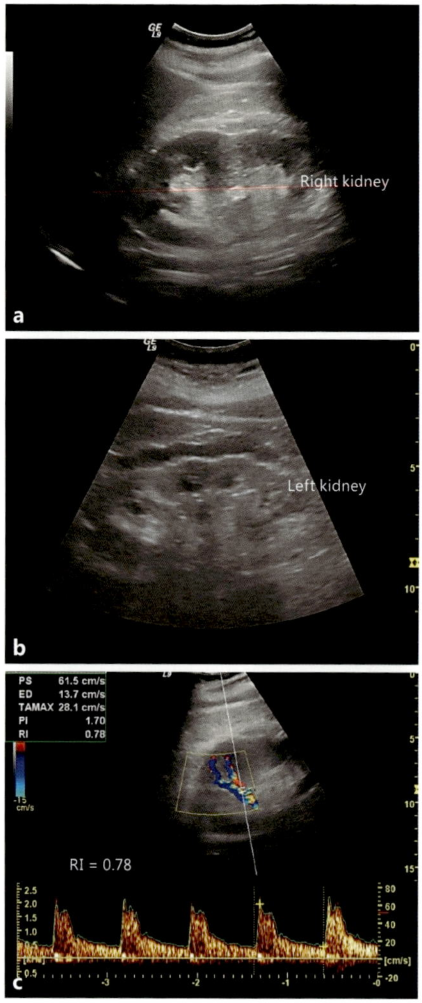

Fig. 2. Post-surgical AKI. Male, aged 66 years, with a functional single kidney. He had a rapid worsening of renal function after colectomy. **a** At B-mode US examination, the right kidney had normal volume (coronal diameter 11.7 cm) and showed a slight hypoechogenicity of mesorenal pyramids. **b** The left kidney was diffusely hyperechoic, with an altered structure and decreased volume (coronal diameter 8.9 cm). **c** At color Doppler sampling of interlobar arteries, renal RIs were increased (0.78). At Doppler sampling of renal arteries, there were no ostial accelerations that may be suggestive of renal artery stenosis.

Actually, evidence demonstrates different renal resistive index (RI) variations on the basis of primary disease. In fact, different diseases may lead to specific pathophysiological variations and subsequent intrarenal hemodynamic changes [6]. In diseases that primarily affect glomerulus, RIs may be normal or low (<0.65); in tubulointerstitial diseases, RIs have intermediate values (between 0.65 and 0.75); while in pathological condition that primarily involve vessels (vasculitis), RIs may be higher than 0.80. In chronic kidney disease (CKD), 0.80 is considered the cutoff value for not recoverable renal failure [7]. In experimental models of glycerol-induced AKI, the prolonged and severe decrease of renal plasma flow was followed by a marked arteriolar vasoconstriction. The subsequent increase in vascular impedance leaded to a rapid rise of RI that achieved

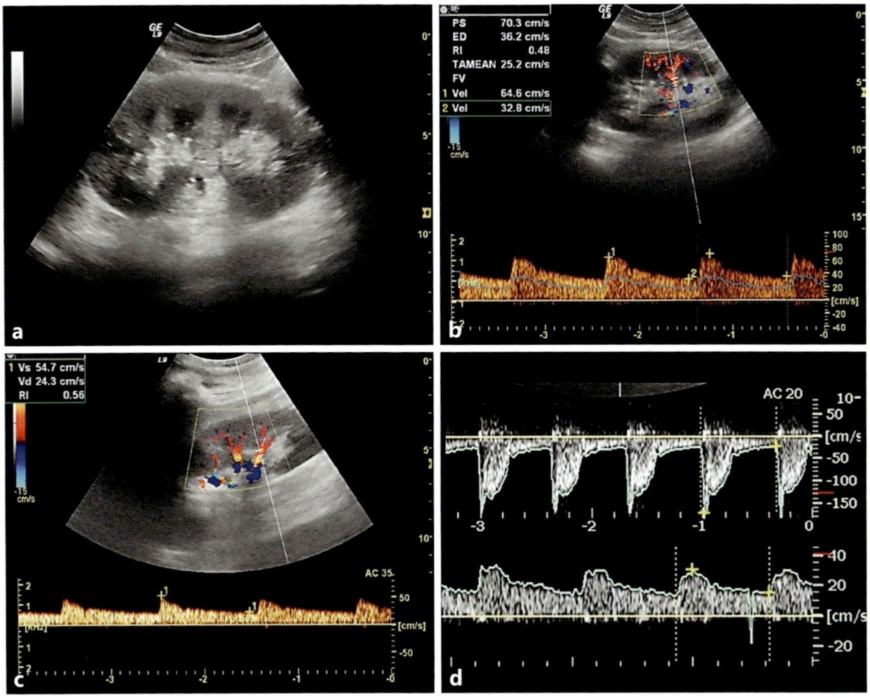

Fig. 3. ATN due to anticryptogamics. Renal recovery phase. Patient of figure 1 underwent renal US and color Doppler after 12 days from the admission in Nephrology Unit. **a** At B-mode US examination, renal morphology was unchanged, while, at color Doppler sampling of interlobar arteries, renal RIs returned to normal values in both the right (**b**) and the left (**c**) kidney. The parenchymal blushing diffusely increased and the diastolic flow was present, indicating low vascular resistances (RI = 0.57–0.59). The recovery of a normal renal perfusion anticipated a moderate polyuric phase, which happened contemporarily to the recovery of renal function. **d** Doppler curves were recorded in the interlobar arteries during the acute phase and the recovery phase.

its peak within 12 h from the induction of AKI. Then, RI progressively returned to normal values in 1 week (fig. 3). Conversely, sCr values reached the peak within the first day and decreased slowly achieving normal values after 2 weeks. Despite RI variation having a linear correlation with sCr increase, it occurred more rapidly, anticipating sCr increase [8]. Since the 1990s, several clinical studies confirmed these experimental data, underlining the utility of RI in diagnosing and characterizing AKI, in different settings. In 1991, Platt et al. [9] showed that in 69% of patients with ATN, intrarenal Doppler US allowed detection of hemodynamic changes associated with AKI and, more interestingly, it was helpful in distinguishing ATN from pre-renal AKI. In fact, in 80% of patients with pre-renal AKI, plasma flow was normal or slightly decreased, with low RI values (<0.65). Conversely, in 91% of patients with ATN, Doppler spectral curve was

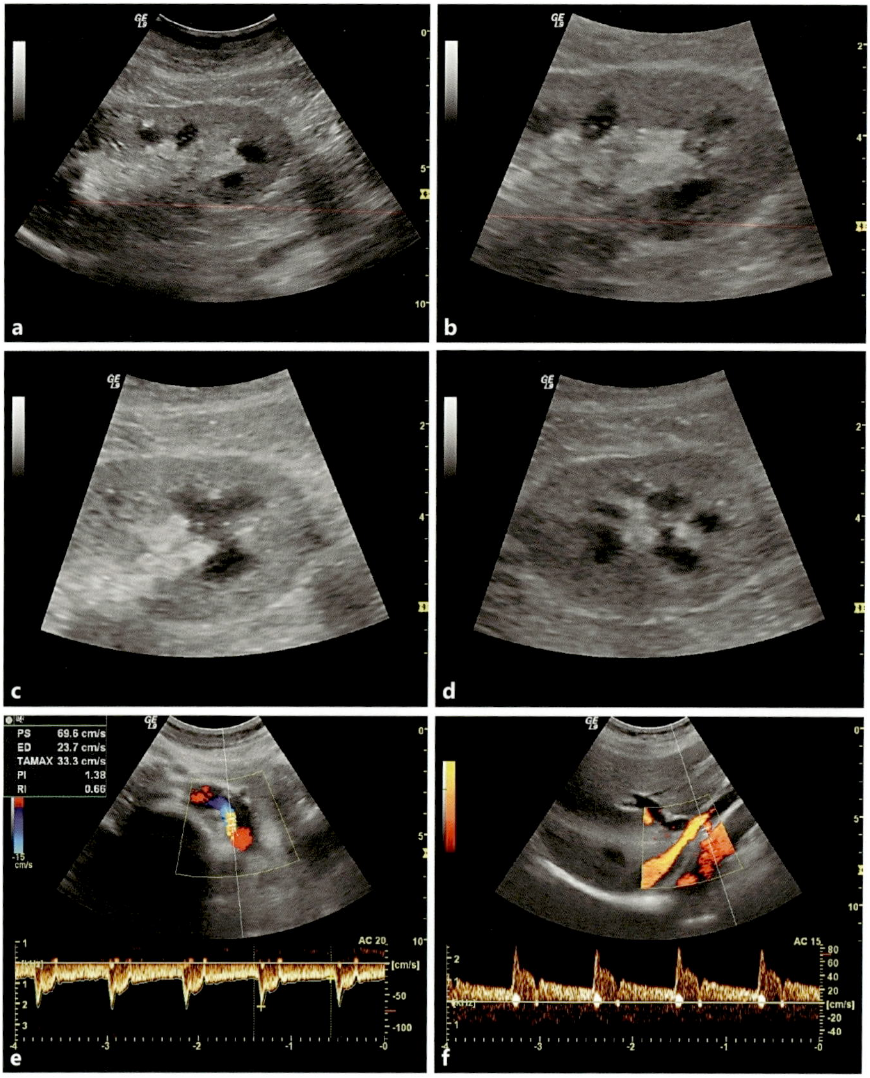

Fig. 4. Acute interstitial nephritis due to non-steroidal anti-inflammatory drugs abuse. The 67-year-old female patient had an acute worsening of renal function (sCr from 1.1 to 2.8 mg/dl). **a**, **b** At B-Mode US examination, kidneys were symmetrical. Coronal diameters were >11 cm and parenchymal thickness was normal, but renal structure was altered. **c**, **d** Cortex appeared diffusely hyperechoic, while medullary pyramids were hypoechoic, well distinguished and with irregular profiles. Corticomedullary alterations became even more evident with a major enlargement. **e**, **f** At color Doppler sampling, renal arteries presented neither direct nor indirect signs of stenosis. Doppler wave showed a high difference between systolic and diastolic phase, because of the decrease of diastolic flow.

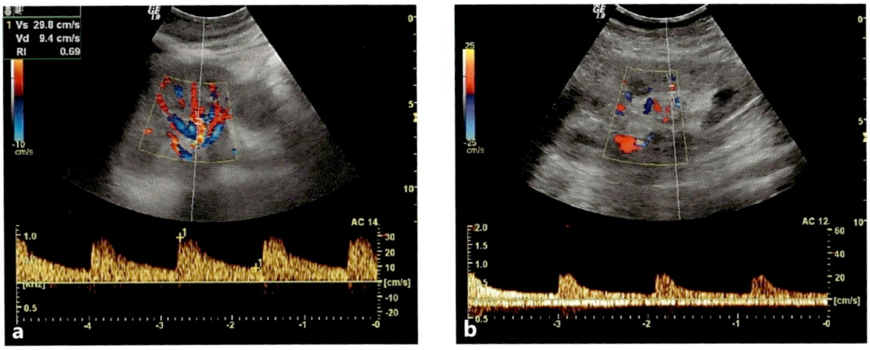

Fig. 5. Acute interstitial nephritis due to non-steroidal anti-inflammatory drug abuse. Parenchymal blushing was well represented. Renal RIs measured in interlobar arteries varied from 0.66 to 0.75. Hemodynamic variations are commonly related to severity and progression of the anatomical damage. **a**, **b** In interstitial nephritis with AKI, potentially recoverable RIs are commonly <0.70.

characterized by the increase of systolic peak velocity and the loss the diastolic flow, leading to a pulsatile flow pattern with RI constantly >0.75. This hemodynamic pattern is clearly explained by the increase of renal vascular impedance [6]. Few years later, the same work group demonstrated that high RI correlated with both delayed renal recovery and requirement of renal replacement therapy [10]. Stevens et al. [11] showed that RIs were also helpful in the early diagnosis of renal recovery. Indeed, the normalization of RI revealed the improvement of renal perfusion and it preceded the decrease of sCr values. Several more recent studies and a meta-analysis confirmed that higher RI values are predictive of persistent AKI [12–14]. Nevertheless, due to the marked heterogeneity among the studies, further investigations focused on timing of RI measurement and test performance are needed.

Acute Interstitial Nephritis

Acute interstitial nephritis is currently a frequent cause of AKI, mainly due to non-steroidal anti-inflammatory drugs (NSAIDs) and antibiotics administration. In addition, it may also occur during systemic immunological diseases, anti-glomerular basement membrane disease and in several systemic infections. The development of acute interstitial nephritis is due to an immunological reaction against nephritogenic exogenous antigens, processed by tubular cells. Acute interstitial nephritis is mainly related to cell-mediated immunity. The inflammatory interstitial infiltration consists of lymphocytes, macrophages, eosinophils and plasma cells and it rapidly evolves to fibrosis. The clinical course is often paucisymptomatic (fever, skin rash, arthralgia, peripheral eosinophilia), and symptoms rapidly improve after the withdrawal of the incriminated drugs. Moreover, recent studies suggest that early administration of corticosteroids (within 7 days from diagnosis) may improve functional recovery and reduce the risk of progression to CKD. Conversely, a delayed steroidal therapy has low beneficial effects [15]. In acute interstitial nephritis, as well as in ATN, conventional US does not allow a definitive diagnosis. Kidneys appear enlarged and widely hyperechoic due to interstitial edema and inflammatory infiltration (fig. 4). In some cases of acute interstitial nephritis related to systemic infection, interstitial edema and infiltration can lead to an acute distention of renal capsule and to a doubling of kidneys volume [16].

At color Doppler, hemodynamic changes are closely correlated to the severity and the progression of the anatomical damage. In fact, in reversible AKI due to acute interstitial nephritis, RIs are commonly ≤0.70 (fig. 5).

References

1 Platt JF, Ellis JH, Rubin JM, DiPietro MA, Sedman AB: Intrarenal arterial Doppler sonography in patients with nonobstructive renal disease: correlation of resistive index with biopsy findings. AJR Am J Roentgenol 1990;154:1223–1227.

2 Sustić A, Mavrić Z, Fuckar Z, Miletić D, Mozetic V, Mlinarić B: Kidney length in postoperative acute renal failure. J Clin Ultrasound 1998;26:251–255.

3 Nomura G, Kinoshita E, Yamagata Y, Koga N: Usefulness of renal ultrasonography for assessment of severity and course of acute tubular necrosis. J Clin Ultrasound 1984;12:135–139.

4 Barozzi L, Valentino M, Santoro A, Mancini E, Pavlica P: Renal ultrasonography in critically ill patients. Crit Care Med 2007;35(5 suppl):S198–S205.

5 Keyserling HF, Fielding JR, Mittelstaedt CA: Renal sonography in the intensive care unit: when is it necessary? J Ultrasound Med 2002;21:517–520.

6 Platt JF, Ellis JH, Rubin JM, DiPietro MA, Sedman AB: Intrarenal arterial Doppler sonography in patients with nonobstructive renal disease: correlation of resistive index with biopsy findings. AJR Am J Roentgenol 1990;154:1223–1227.

7 Radermacher J, Ellis S, Haller H: Renal resistance index and progression of renal disease. Hypertension 2002;39(2 pt 2):699–703.

8 Yoon D, Kim SH, Kim HD, Na DG, Goo JM, Choi HJ, Yeon KM, Han MC: Doppler sonography in experimentally induced acute renal failure in rabbits. Resistive index versus serum creatinine levels. Invest Radiol 1995;30:168–172.

9 Platt J, Rubin JM, Ellis JH: Acute renal failure: possible role of duplex Doppler US in distinction between acute prerenal failure and acute tubular necrosis. Radiology 1991;179:419–423.

10 Platt JF: Doppler ultrasound of the kidney. Semin Ultrasound CT MR 1997;18:22–32.

11 Stevens PE, Gwyther SJ, Hanson ME, Boultbee JE, Kox WJ, Phillips ME: Noninvasive monitoring of renal blood flow characteristics during acute renal failure in man. Intensive Care Med 1990;16:153–158.

12 Darmon M, Schortgen F, Vargas F, Liazydi A, Schlemmer B, Brun-Buisson C, Brochard L: Diagnostic accuracy of Doppler renal resistive index for reversibility of acute kidney injury in critically ill patients. Intensive Care Med 2011;37:68–76.

13 Bossard G, Bourgoin P, Corbeau JJ, Huntzinger J, Beydon L: Early detection of postoperative acute kidney injury by Doppler renal resistive index in cardiac surgery with cardiopulmonary bypass. Br J Anaesth 2011;107: 891–898.
14 Guinot PG, Bernard E, Abou Arab O, Badoux L, Diouf M, Zogheib E, Dupont H: Doppler-based renal resistive index can assess progression of acute kidney injury in patients undergoing cardiac surgery. J Cardiothorac Vasc Anesth 2013;27:890–896.
15 Praga M, González E: Acute interstitial nephritis. Kidney Int 2010;77:956–961.
16 Hiraoka M, Hori C, Tsuchida S, Tsukahara H, Sudo M: Ultrasonographic findings of acute tubulointerstitial nephritis. Am J Nephrol 1996;16:154–158.

Claudio Ronco, MD
Director of Department of Nephrology Dialysis and Transplantation
International Renal Research Institute (IRRIV), San Bortolo Hospital
Viale Rodolfi 37, IT–36100 Vicenza (Italy)
E-Mail cronco@goldnet.it

Meola M, Petrucci I, Ronco C (eds): Ultrasound Imaging in Acute and Chronic Kidney Disease.
Contrib Nephrol. Basel, Karger, 2016, vol 188, pp 48–63 (DOI: 10.1159/000445467)

Clinical Scenarios in Acute Kidney Injury-Parenchymal Acute Kidney Injury – Vascular Diseases

Mario Meola[a, b] · Sara Samoni[a, c] · Ilaria Petrucci[a, b] · Claudio Ronco[c]

[a]Sant'Anna School of Advanced Studies, Pisa, [b]Department of Internal Medicine, University of Pisa, Pisa, and [c]Department of Nephrology Dialysis and Transplantation, International Renal Research Institute (IRRIV), San Bortolo Hospital, Vicenza, Italy

Abstract

Acute cortical necrosis and hemolytic uremic syndrome (HUS) are 2 clinical scenarios of parenchymal acute kidney injury (AKI) related to renal microvascular injury. Acute cortical necrosis is a rare condition related to an ischemic necrosis of renal cortex. Necrotic lesions can be due to several injuries and may be focal, multifocal or diffuse. Renal necrotic lesions become visible with ultrasound only after renal recovery. HUS is a rare disease characterized by hemolytic anemia, thrombocytopenia and AKI. Color Doppler ultrasound is useful during diagnostic and follow-up phase. Renal artery thrombosis and renal vein thrombosis may also cause parenchymal AKI. Acute renal infarction is a rare pathological condition that occurs due to clots or cholesterol aggregates occluding renal artery or its branches. Several causes may lead to partial or massive kidney ischemic necrosis. Contrast-enhanced CT allows definitive diagnosis in 80% of cases and, at present, it is the first imaging technique used. Ultrasound (US) sensitivity and specificity significantly increases with color Doppler and contrast-enhanced US (CEUS). In AKI patients, in whom the use of iodinated contrast media is contraindicated, color Doppler and CEUS may be valid alternatives for the diagnosis of acute renal infarction. Renal vein thrombosis may be primary or secondary to retroperitoneal neoplasm or inflammatory diseases. It rarely causes an acute worsening of renal function because of the presence of several anastomosis that prevent parenchymal necrosis due to venous congestion. Color Doppler US could detect thrombus within the lumen and document the absence of venous flow.

Introduction

Acute renal microvascular damage is a parenchymal cause of acute kidney injury (AKI). It may be classified as follows: (1) immunological diseases, such as rapidly progressive glomerulonephritis, vasculitis, kidney rejection; (2) degenerative diseases, such as malignant hypertension; (3) hematological diseases, such as hemolytic uremic syndrome (HUS), thrombotic thrombocytopenic purpura and disseminated intravascular coagulation.

Renal artery thrombosis and renal vein thrombosis are also responsible for parenchymal AKI related to renal vascular diseases.

Acute Cortical Necrosis

Acute cortical necrosis is a rare cause of AKI. It is related to an ischemic necrosis of renal cortex. Necrotic lesions can be due to arterial vasospasm, microvascular damage, drugs administration or disseminated intravascular coagulation. Necrosis may be delimited and multifocal or may involve the entire cortex of both kidneys. This last condition is rare and it is due to shock, sepsis, acute myocardial infarction or burns. In most cases, medulla, juxtamedullary cortex and a thin layer of sub-capsular cortex are not damaged. Morphological and structural characteristics of kidneys in cortical necrosis are inconstant. During the acute phase of diffuse acute cortical necrosis, renal ultrasound (US) shows kidneys with normal volume, with no differentiation between cortex and medulla and, occasionally, a thin hypoechoic peri-renal layer related to reactive edema [1]. Acute cortical necrosis may also be related to intense physical activity. It can be due to rhabdomyolysis and subsequent myoglobinuria, or due to anaerobic exercise, with neither myoglobinuria nor type II fiber myolysis [2]. According to several literature reports, the last clinical condition could be due to the administration of non-steroidal anti-inflammatory drugs (NSAIDs) and arterial hypotension, and it is characterized by severe back pain after intense physical activity. In these cases, renal US shows wedge-shaped hypoechoic areas, which are extended from the cortex to the medulla. Renal necrotic lesions are detectable by CT since the onset phase of AKI, while they become visible with US only after renal recovery (fig. 1) [3]. Contrast-enhanced US (CEUS) may improve the diagnosis of diffuse acute cortical necrosis. Otherwise, due to the rarity of this disease and the critical conditions of patients affected, literature evidence is missing.

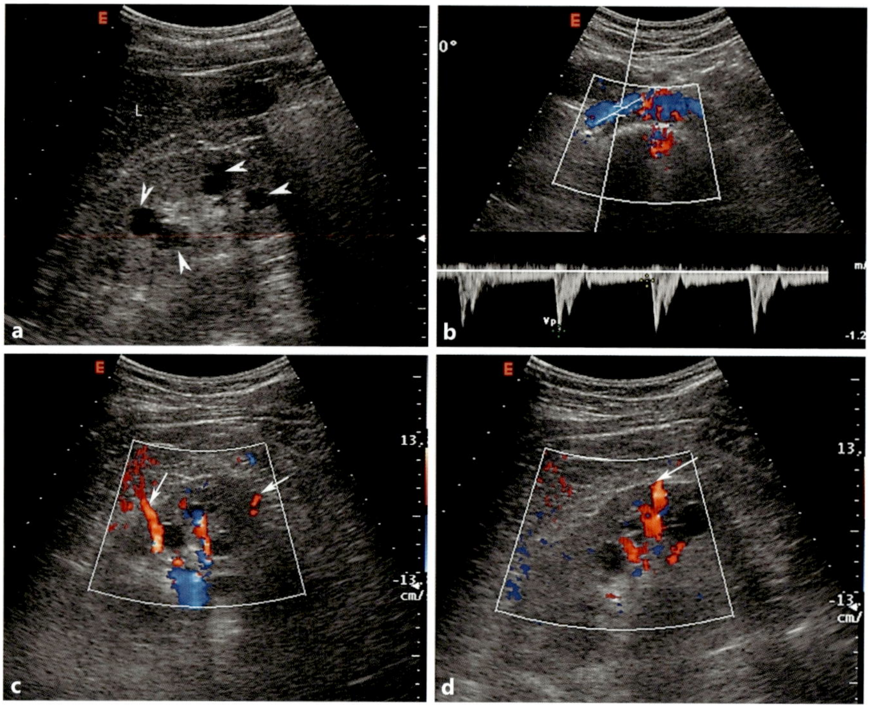

Fig. 1. Acute cortical necrosis. Male, aged 38 years. Intense physical activity and food supplements/creatine abuse. After intense physical activity in bad weather conditions and use of NSAIDs for fever, he developed acute worsening of renal function, arterial hypotension and severe lumbar pain without myoglobinuria. Since there was no renal recovery, patient started chronic hemodialysis. One month later, conventional US showed (**a**) kidneys with decreased volume (coronal diameter 9 cm), hyperechoic parenchyma with multiple hypoechoic gaps (arrowheads) diffused in both cortex and medulla. **b** Renal artery showed a Doppler wave with increased resistances and diastolic flow still present. **c**, **d** Color Doppler sampling showed several transcapsular vessels with flow toward perirenal space (arrow). L = Liver.

Hemolytic Uremic Syndrome

HUS is a rare disease characterized by hemolytic anemia, thrombocytopenia and AKI. In children, HUS is the most common cause of AKI, and in most cases, it achieves full renal recovery without any clinical consequences. In adults, HUS is rarer than in children and it has a worse course, thus possibly leading to irreversible chronic kidney disease (CKD) and death. The etiology of HUS is still debated. Otherwise, in most cases, it occurs after severe gastrointestinal infections due to ingestion of water or foods, such as undercooked meat or milk products, contaminated with Escherichia coli or Shigella

Dyssenteriae [4]. Enterobacteria release toxins into the circulation causing a severe endothelial damage to capillaries and arterioles of both kidneys and brain. Nevertheless, the neurological damage is more important in thrombotic thrombocytopenic purpura than in HUS. In the most severe cases, verotoxins released by enterobacteria can also impair mucosal vessels of bowel, leading to hemorrhagic colitis. Thickening of vessel wall, due to endothelial cells swelling and detachment, and thrombosis of microvessels are the most common histopathological signs of HUS. Kidney lesions are different on the basis of the age of patients with HUS. In children up to 2 years, lesions are primarily localized into glomeruli. In children over 2 years and in adults, glomerular injury is more variable, while signs of thrombotic microangiopathy of renal arteries and arterioles and post-glomerular capillaries are prevalent. The presence of neurological symptoms, which is related to the damage of small cerebral arteries, negatively influences patient outcomes. HUS can also have an unusual clinical course. Severe HUS is characterized by hemorrhagic colitis, rapidly progressive kidney failure and resistant hypertension. Less severe HUS does not cause diarrhea during early stages and cause progressive renal insufficiency that develops in parallel with neurological symptoms onset. A particular type of HUS affects several family members, thus indicating a genetic predisposition rather than a common exposure to the same cause. In addition, HUS can occur in pregnancy or be related to drug administration [5], malignancy or HIV infection.

US in HUS shows enlarged kidneys with well-defined and hypoechoic pyramids and a diffusely hyperechoic cortex. During the acute phase, as vasoconstriction leads to the development of thrombotic microangiopathy, Doppler wave shows a decrease of diastolic flow in renal artery and an important increase of renal resistive indexes (RIs). In the most severe conditions, Doppler wave may show a reverse flow [6]. Morphological and Doppler parameters progressively achieve normal values parallel to renal recovery. Nevertheless, 5 years after the resolution of HUS, RIs are still significantly superior to age-matched healthy subjects [6–8].

Renal Artery Thrombosis

Acute renal infarction is a rare pathological condition that occurs due to clots or cholesterol aggregates that move into circulation leading to the obstruction of renal artery or its branches. In about 50% of cases, emboli derive from the breakdown of a left atrial thrombus during atrial fibrillation. In other cases, thromboembolism is primitive and occurs in young subjects without any thrombogenic risk factor [9]. Cholesterol emboli move from spontaneous or iatrogenic fragmentation of an aortic calcified plaque. Ischemic necrosis can be partial (focal or multifocal) or massive (mono or bilateral). Most cases of partial or segmental infarction are related to embolism during atrial fibrillation or endocarditis (fig. 2) [10]. Rarely, acute renal infarction is due to spontaneous dissection of renal artery (fig. 3), dilated cardiomyopathy [11] and paradoxical embolism. In about 10% of cases, both kidneys are affected. Usually, bilateral renal infarction is related to aortic injury or surgery [12] (fig. 4). More rare conditions associated to bilateral renal infarction are aortic dissection, septic emboli during endocarditis, systemic lupus erythematosus, vasculitis secondary to sickle cell disease [13], antiphospholipid antibody syndrome [14] and cocaine abuse [15].

Kidneys are not frequently affected by peripheral arterial thromboembolism. In a study that enrolled more than 600 patients, the arteries most frequently affected by thromboembolism were lower limbs arteries (61%), mesenteric arteries (29%), pelvic arteries (9%), aorta (7%) and, lastly, renal arteries (2%) [16]. Renal thromboembolism mostly affects adult-elderly subjects (age >65 years) of both gender.

The onset is characterized by intense lumbar or abdominal pain, fever, nausea and vomit. Rarely, acute renal infarction begins with arterial hypertension or oliguria and AKI. During the emergency phase, differential diagnosis may be very difficult. All causes of acute surgical abdomen must be excluded (appendicitis, diverticulitis, ruptured abdominal aortic aneurysm, testicular/ovarian torsion, strangulated hernia, intestinal obstruction and/or perforation), as well as acute non-surgical causes (mesenteric ischemia, nephrolithiasis, pyelonephritis). In this phase, the diagnosis is possible only in 40% of patients, while in other cases acute renal infarction is unrecognized (fig. 5). Hematuria is frequently, but not constantly present. On the contrary, increase of LDH and leukocytosis are always present. Proteinuria occurs in only 45% of patients, while C-reactive protein is often increased. Renal function may be normal. Nevertheless, when necrosis is extensive, AKI occurs [17].

The most common consequences of acute renal infarction are renal function loss and resistant arterial hypertension. Many patients undergo CKD and in few cases (8%) renal replacement therapy is required [18].

Angiography is considered the gold standard for the diagnosis of renal artery thrombosis, with a sensitivity of 100%. Renal scintigraphy is positive in 97% of cases. Contrast-enhanced CT is positive in 80% of cases and, at present, it is the first imaging technique used. US is rarely useful for definitive diagnosis (3% of cases), although its sensitivity and specificity significantly increase with color Doppler and CEUS. In contrast-enhanced CT, renal parenchyma

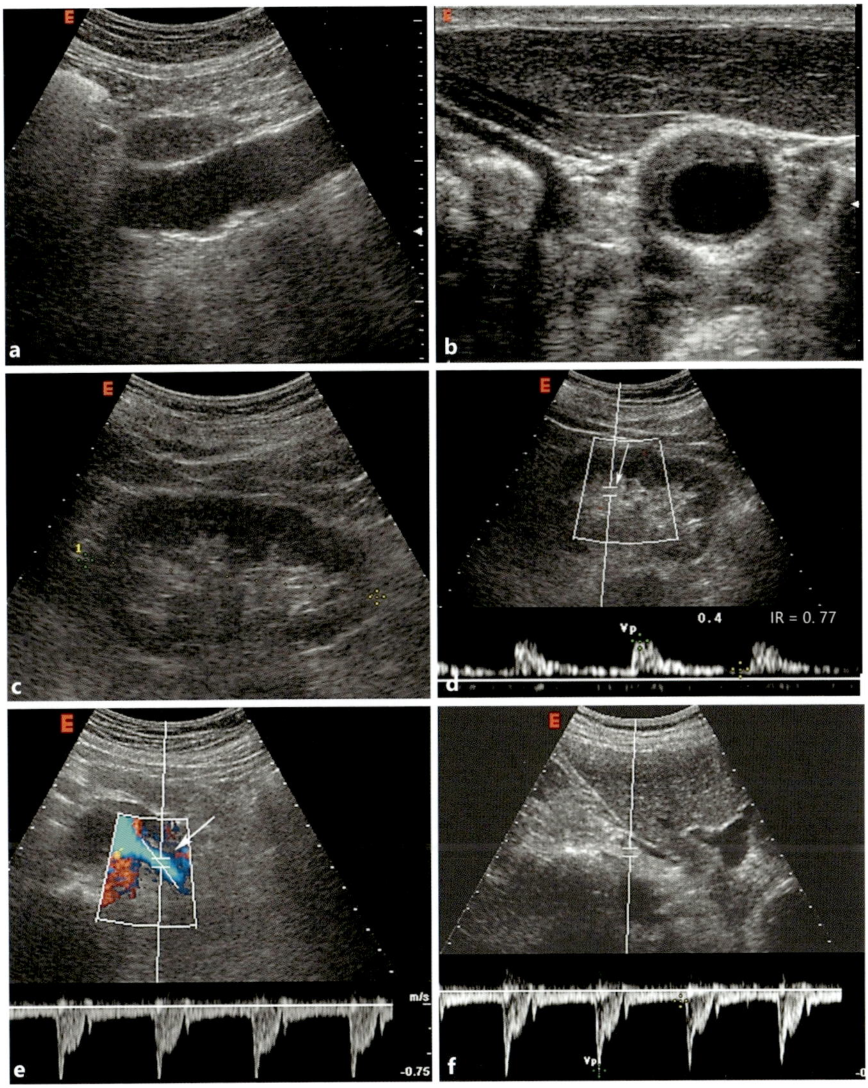

Fig. 2. AKI due to iatrogenic atheroembolism. Female, aged 65 years. After a diagnostic arteriography, patient had a rapid worsening of renal function with an increase of serum creatinine (from 1.6 to 6.6 mg/dl), eosinophilia (8.5%), LDH 375 UI/l. **a** At B-mode US evaluation, aorta showed mild atheromasia. **b** Carotid arteries showed severe atheromasia. **c** Abdominal B-Mode examination showed normal kidneys volume and sinus sclerolipomatosis. Right kidney had decreased parenchymal thickness. **d** Color Doppler sampling of interlobular arteries showed high renal RIs (0.77–0.81). **e**, **f** Color Doppler sampling of renal arteries excluded stenosis. Doppler wave with an important systo-diastolic difference was indicative of increased intraparenchymal vascular resistances.

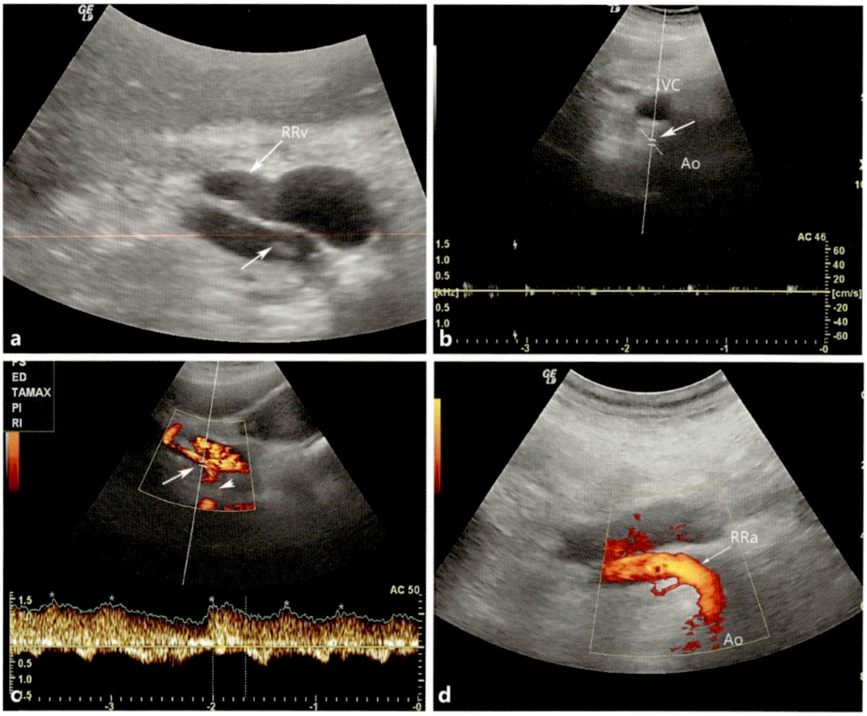

Fig. 3. AKI due to arterial thromboembolism in single kidney patient. A 78-year-old male with severe systemic arteriopathy (previous acute myocardial infarction, aortocoronary bypass, aorto-bisiliac graft, obliterative arterial disease of the lower limbs, previous transient ischemic attacks), atrial fibrillation and previous left nephrectomy due to neoplasm. His baseline serum creatinine (sCr) was 1.6 mg/dl. He was referred to the nephrologist because of rapid worsening of renal function (sCr up to 10.9 mg/dl) and anuria. US examination excluded vesical globus and atrial thrombus. The right kidney appeared globose-shaped (coronal diameter 13 cm), diffusely hypoechoic and with poor vascularization. **a** US B-mode examination showed hypoechoic material into the renal artery at the ostium, with floating intimal flap (arrow). **b** At color Doppler sampling, there was no signal at the ostium. **c** Collateral vessels (white arrow) perfused distal main renal artery, which had an ostial stenosis (arrowhead). (*) Spectral analysis showed slow blood flow secondary to atrial arrhythmia. The patient refused arteriography. He started hemodialysis and thrombolysis with continuous infusion of heparin for 5 days. **d** At color Doppler, after 10 days from the withdrawal of heparin, artery became patent. Doppler wave at ostium (**e**) and at hilum (**f**) did not show signals of stenosis. Intraparenchymal renal RIs were 0.76. Patient was discharged with anticoagulant therapy (sCr 1.8 mg/dl). RRv = Right renal vein; IVC = inferior vena cava; Ao = aorta; RRa = right renal artery.

(*For figure 3e and f see next page.*)

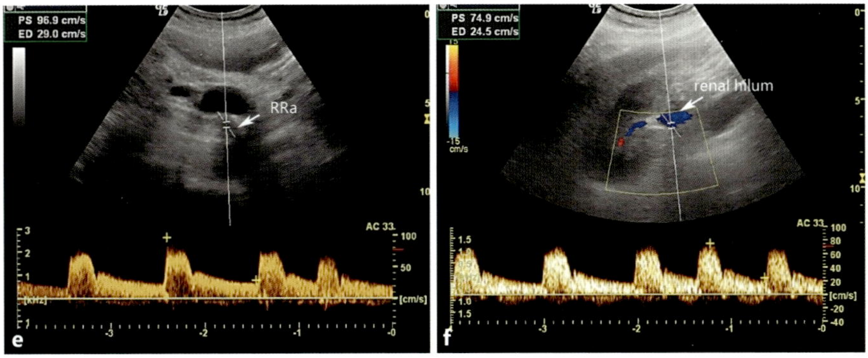

3

affected by ischemic necrosis appears hypodense, wedge-shaped from renal medulla to cortex and it is not enhanced with contrast media. In addition, necrotic area is delimited by a thin hyperdense outline, which is the thin subcortical parenchymal layer, perfused by capsular arteries [19]. This hyperdense outline allows differential diagnosis between ischemic lesion (especially if it is extensive) and pyelonephritic area, in which the outline is usually missed. When CT scan is negative, but LDH increases, patient should be monitored. In this case, a renal scintigraphy is indicated to evaluate potential occurrence of sclerotic areas.

In patients with AKI, the use of iodinated contrast media is contraindicated. In this setting, CT sensitivity decreases and CEUS may be a valid alternative for the diagnosis of acute renal infarction. It should be performed with low mechanical index sonographic contrast media and dedicated color power Doppler sequences using second harmonic imaging and pulse inversion [20, 21].

In acute massive renal thrombosis, color Doppler allows an immediate diagnosis. Kidney is enlarged, globose-shaped, hypoechoic and not perfused. The absence of vascular signal persists even after contrast media administration. On the contrary, segmental renal infarction appears as a hypoechoic and non-perfused triangular area. This aspect characterizes both focal ischemic necrosis and focal pyelonephritis, in which hypoperfusion is due to massive infiltration of inflammatory cells. Contrast media administration improves the evaluation of small vessels (Ø <400 μm), thus identifying focal or multifocal ischemic areas with higher sensitivity. Nevertheless, without a clear clinical setting, CEUS does not allow differential diagnosis. The reliability of color Doppler and CEUS are often limited by technical and anatomical problems. For instance, small subcortical or polar infarction is difficult to diagnose in native kidney, as well as in kidney transplant. Moreover, the low frequency of renal artery thrombosis and the

4

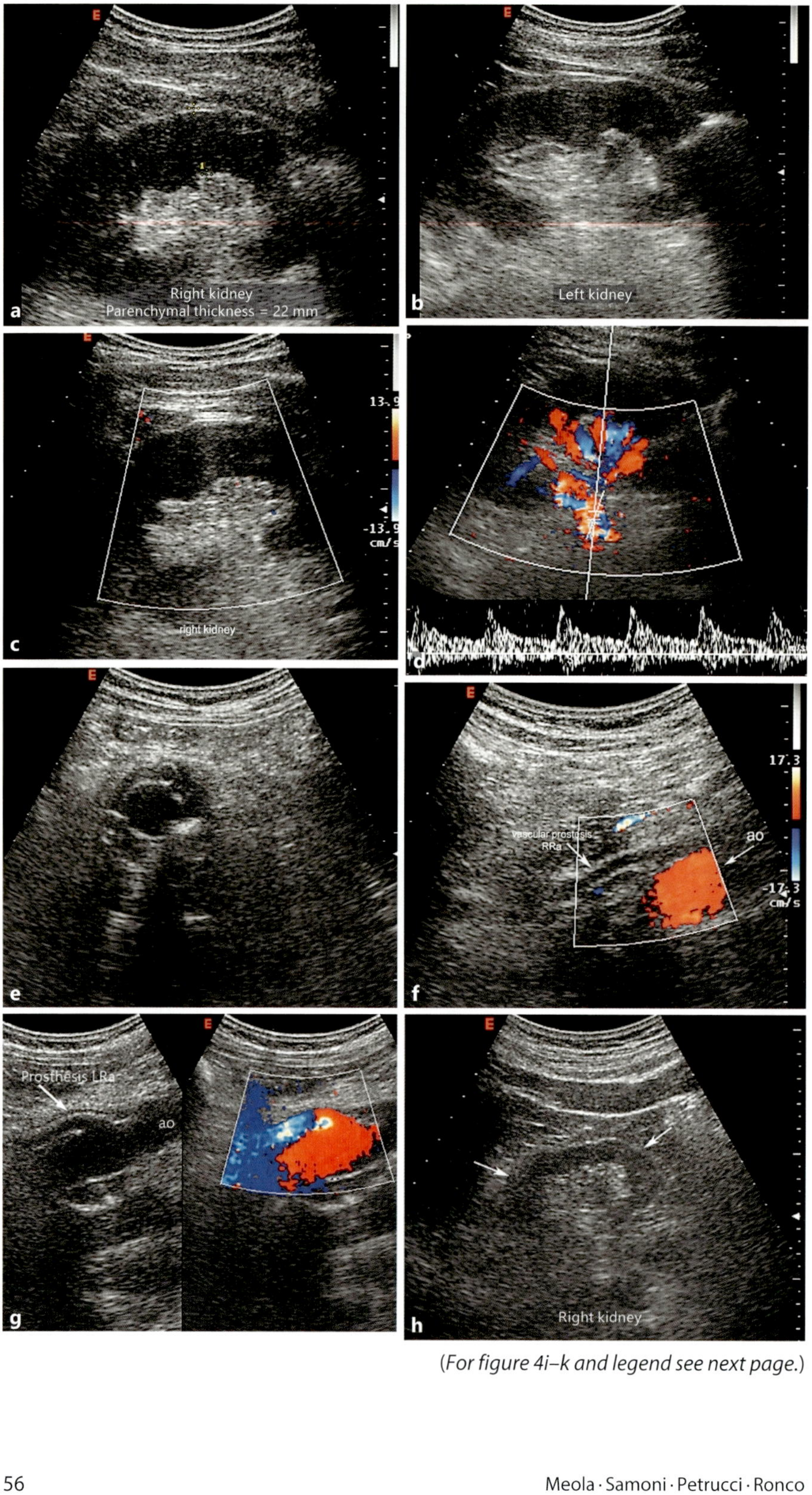

(*For figure 4i–k and legend see next page.*)

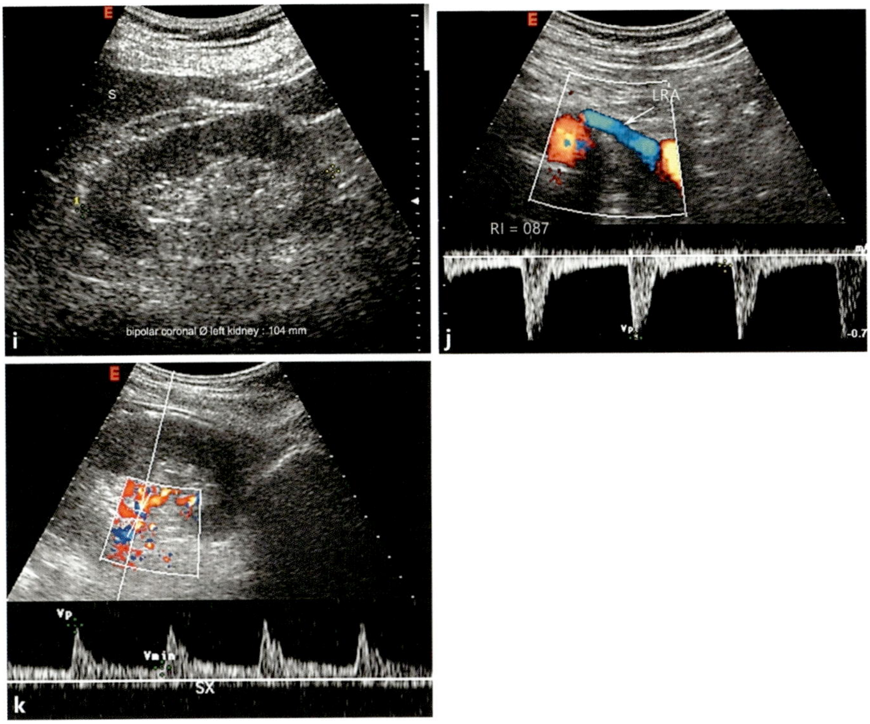

Fig. 4. Acute thrombosis of right renal artery. Male, aged 68 years, with systemic arteriopathy and pararenal aortic aneurysm treated with conventional aneurismorraffy and reimplantation of renal arteries into the graft after fissuration. After surgery, patient had renal recovery and his baseline serum creatinine (sCr) was 1.7 mg/dl. One month after surgical intervention and after heparin withdrawal, he had a rapid worsening of renal function (sCr 8,4 mg/dl) with oliguria and a severe lumbar pain. **a**, **b** At B-Mode examination, kidneys were enlarged and globose-shaped (coronal diameter >12.5 cm). Right kidney was hypoechoic compared to left kidney. **c** At color Doppler sampling, the right kidney was not perfused, while (**d**) the left kidney had a normal vascularization. **e** Aortic and renal grafts were surrounded by reactive tissue. **f** At color-Doppler sampling, vascular prosthesis of right renal artery was not perfused, while (**g**) the left renal artery prosthesis had a normal vascularization. Arteriography was not performed. Patient underwent medical thrombolysis. One month after acute renal artery thrombosis, sCr was stable (2.3–2.8 mg/dl). At B-Mode examination, right kidney was athrophic (coronal diameter <6 cm) (**h**), while left kidney was normal (coronal diameter 10.4 cm) (**i**). Left renal artery was patent and Doppler wave showed a decreased diastolic flow (**j**) due to the increase of intraparenchymal renal RIs (**k**). RRa = Right renal artery.

lack of studies on large series do not allow considering CEUS as the first examination in the management of these patients. The more frequent use of CEUS may indicate, in the future, the precise role of this technique in the diagnosis of renal infarction.

Renal Vein Thrombosis

Renal vein thrombosis may occur in renal and/or retroperitoneal cancer, perirenal abscesses, trauma, compression by aberrant arterial vessels or it may be related to primary renal diseases with nephrotic syndrome. Primary renal vein thrombosis is classified into 2 clinical variants: (1) renal vein thrombosis in newborns and in children, characterized by dehydration and subsequent hypercoagulability and thrombocytopenia [22] and (2) renal vein thrombosis related to nephrotic syndrome, in adults [23] (fig. 6).

Renal vein thrombosis rarely causes an acute worsening of renal function because of the presence of several intrarenal and para-renal anastomosis that prevent parenchymal necrosis due to venous congestion. However, in the case of acute renal vein occlusion (10% of cases), collateral vessels cannot prevent an acute venous congestion. This leads to an increase in kidney volume, a decrease in renal blood flow and, subsequently, to AKI. On the contrary, total or partial renal vein thrombosis may be paucisymptomatic if it develops sub-acutely or chronically.

Fig. 5. Renal infarction due to thromboembolism of anterior branch of the right renal artery. A 43-year-old female was referred to nephrologist because of CKD stage 2 and suspicious of chronic pyelonephritis. **a, b** At B-mode examination, right kidney appeared small, sclero-atrophic, with normal posterior parenchyma. **c** Right renal artery had a slow flow characterized by low resistances. **d** Color Doppler sampling of right segmental posterior artery showed a low resistance flow with renal RI of 0.58. Left renal artery (**e**) and left intrarenal arteries (**f**) were normal. Patient's anamnesis reported several untreated episodes of tachyarrhythmia. The main episode occurred when patient was 27 years old. It was accompanied by acute and severe right lumbar pain and *de-novo* arterial hypertension. Blood pressure returned spontaneously to normal values after 2 years. Serum creatinine (sCr) was normal. Diagnostic hypothesis was renal infarction due to thromboembolism of anterior branch of the right renal artery. Separate renal function measured by renal scintigraphy (Gates method) confirmed the right kidney decreased function (creatinine clearance – CrCl- 26 ml/min) and left kidney normal function (CrCl 75 ml/min). This clinical case demonstrates that renal infarction is often misdiagnosed. RRa = Right renal artery.

(*For figure see next page.*)

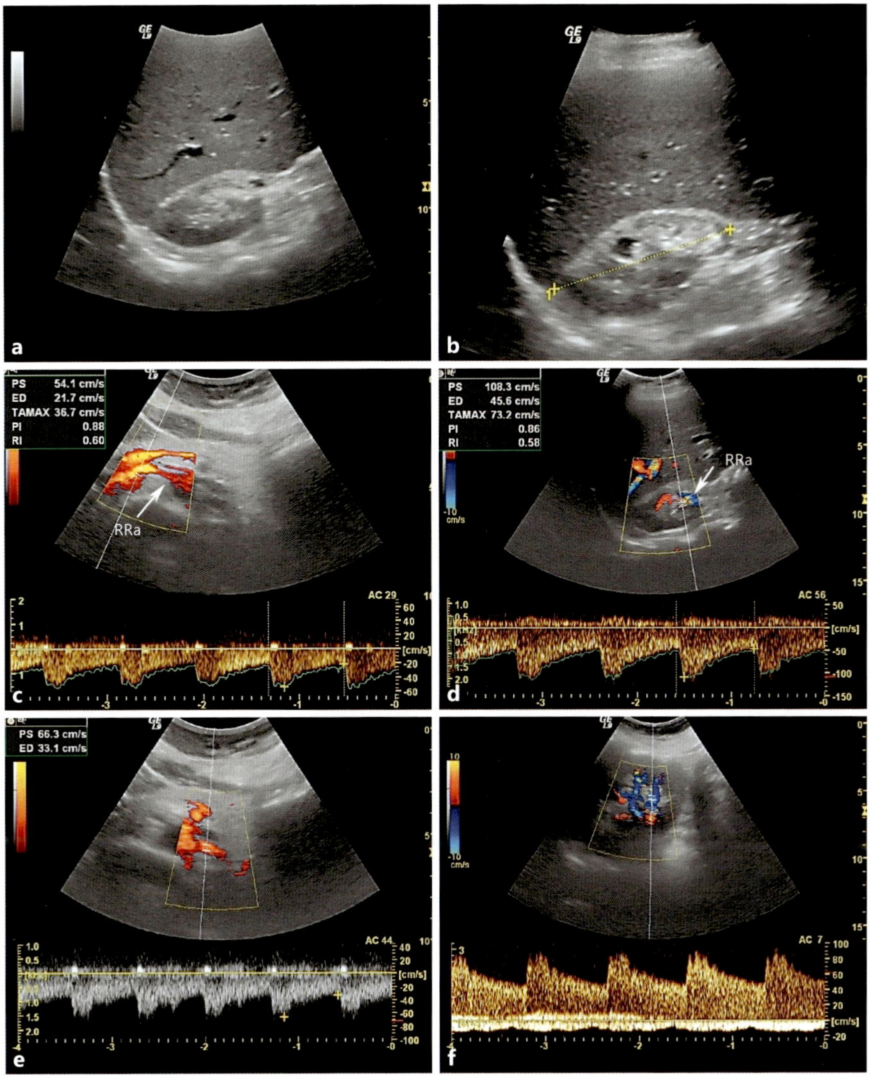

5

US and color Doppler findings are (1) visualization of iso-echogenic (recent thrombosis) or hyper-echogenic organized thrombus within renal vein, which occupies part of or the entire lumen; (2) absent or decreased venous flow; (3) absent velocity/time curve in renal vein [24].

An important sign allows differentiating primary from secondary renal vein thrombosis: in primary diseases, thrombi occupy the entire vein lumen but do not deform it, while in secondary diseases, renal vein appears irregular and dilated due to thrombus wall compression [25].

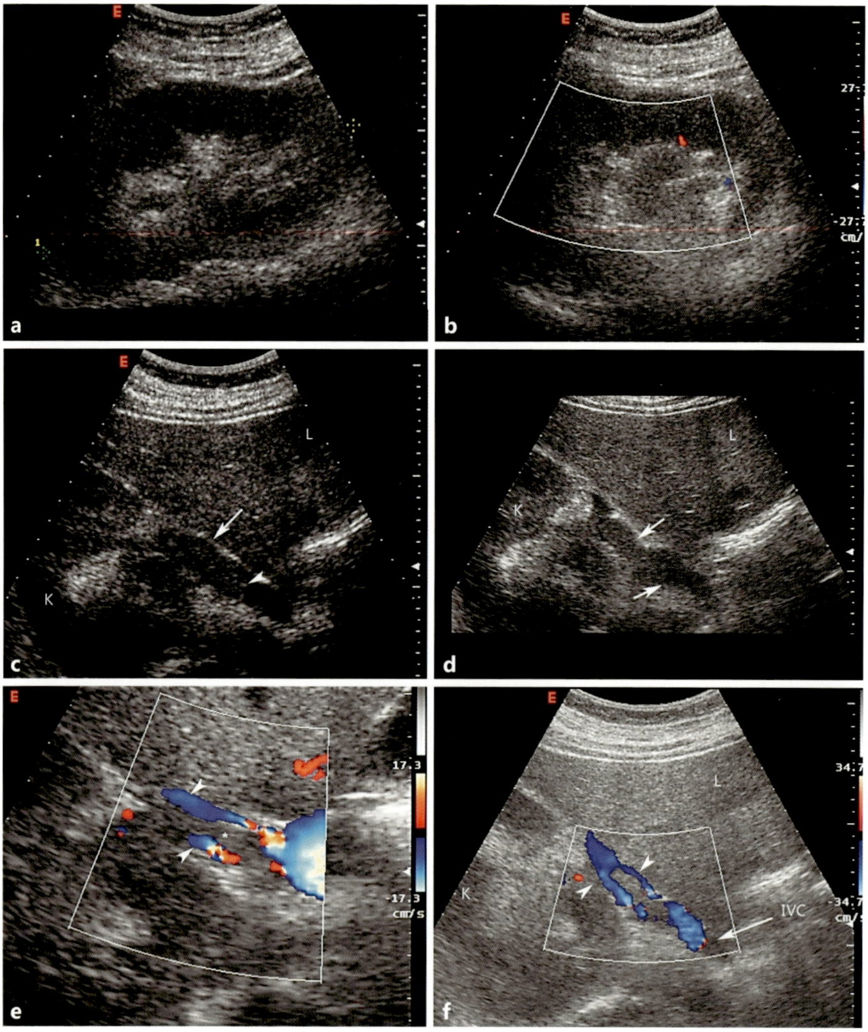

Fig. 6. Bilateral renal vein thrombosis in a patient with nephritic syndrome secondary to focal glomerulosclerosis. Male, aged 23 years, with normal glomerular filtration rate (GFR) and proteinuria 12–17 g/day. US evaluation was required after acute worsening of GFR and low back pain (serum creatinine was 3.7 mg/dl). **a** Right kidney longitudinal diameter was 14 cm and it appeared hypoechoic, globose-shaped and hypoperfused (**b**). RI was 0.68. **c**, **d** Right renal vein showed a hypoechoic material (white arrows) filling most part of the lumen (arrowhead). After systemic anticoagulant therapy (**e**, **f**) vein showed a partial recanalization with thin flow signals (arrowhead) around the thrombus. The progressive improvement in vessel perfusion occurred together with functional recovery. K = Kidney; L = liver; IVC = inferior vena cava.

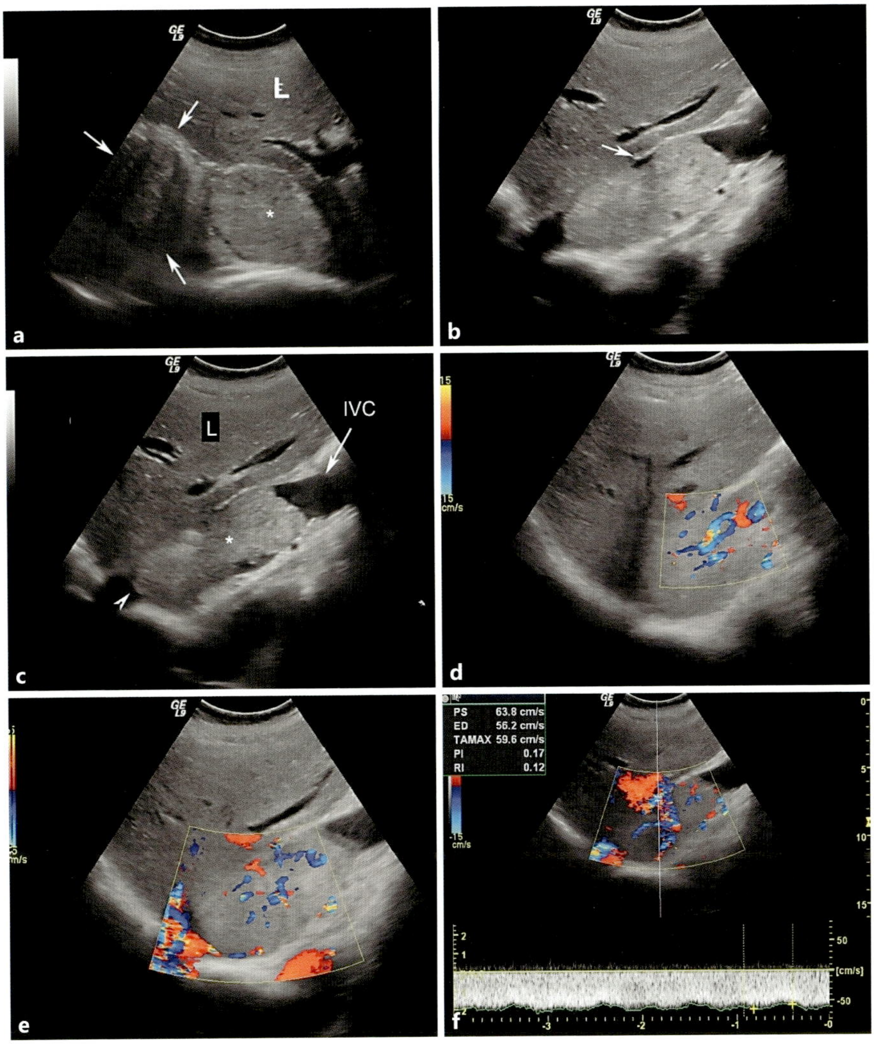

Fig. 7. Neoplastic thrombosis of right renal vein and inferior vena cava. **a** Ascending subcostal right scan shows a non-homogeneous hypoechoic renal mass of the upper lip of the right renal sinus (white arrows). A round hyperechoic mass fills the lumen of the inferior vena cava (*). **b**, **c** Paramedian sagittal scan on intrahepatic vena cava. Inferior vena cava is occupied by a solid hyperechoic nodule (arrow), which enlarges the vein without occluding it. Thrombosis extent (arrowhead) is toward sub-diaphragmatic inferior vena cava (caval thrombosis level II). **d**, **e** Caval thrombus shows a rich and irregular vascular network. **f** Spectral analysis shows thin flow signals around the thrombus profile. L = Liver; IVC = inferior vena cava.

References

1 Sefczek RJ, Beckman I, Lupetin AR, Dash N: Sonography of acute renal cortical necrosis. AJR Am J Roentgenol 1984;142:553–554.

2 Ishikawa I: Acute renal failure with severe loin pain and patchy renal ischemia after anaerobic exercise in patients with or without renal hypouricemia. Nephron 2002;91:559–570.

3 Sakemi T, Ikeda Y, Matsuo Y, Kudo S, Nishihara G, Baba N: Renal wedge-shaped lesions on computed tomography and ultrasonography in two patients who developed acute renal failure with severe loin pain after exercise. Nephron 1996;73:679–681.

4 Matsell DG, White CT: An outbreak of diarrhea-associated childhood hemolytic uremic syndrome: the Walkerton epidemic. Kidney Int Suppl 2009;112:S35–S37.

5 Al-nouri ZL, Reese JA, Terrell DR, Vesely SK, George JN: Drug-induced thrombotic microangiopathy: a systematic review of published reports. Blood 2015;125:616–618.

6 Lemmer A, Bergmann K, Walch R, Endert G: [Doppler ultrasound studies of long-term follow-up of children with hemolytic-uremic syndrome]. Ultraschall Med 1995;16:127–131.

7 Glatstein M, Miller E, Garcia-Bournissen F, Scolnik D: Timing and utility of ultrasound in diarrhea-associated hemolytic uremic syndrome: 7-year experience of a large tertiary care hospital. Clin Pediatr (Phila) 2010;49: 418–421.

8 Capotondo L, Nicolai GA, Garosi G: The role of color Doppler in acute kidney injury. Arch Ital Urol Androl 2010;82:275–279.

9 Bolderman R, Oyen R, Verrijcken A, Knockaert D, Vanderschueren S: Idiopathic renal infarction. Am J Med 2006;119:356.e9–e12.

10 Paris B, Bobrie G, Rossignol P, Le Coz S, Chedid A, Plouin PF: Blood pressure and renal outcomes in patients with kidney infarction and hypertension. J Hypertens 2006;24: 1649–1654.

11 Can MM, Tanboğa IH, Demircan HC, Ozkan A, Koca F, Keleş N, Sönmez K, Kaymaz C, Serebruany V: Acute kidney infarction secondary to intracardiac thrombus embolization in a patient with ischemic dilated cardiomyopathy. Cardiology 2010;117:219–221.

12 Tsai SH, Chu SJ, Chen SJ, Fan YM, Chang WC, Wu CP, Hsu CW: Acute renal infarction: a 10-year experience. Int J Clin Pract 2007;61:62–67.

13 Granfortuna J, Zamkoff K, Urrutia E: Acute renal infarction in sickle cell disease. Am J Hematol 1986;23:59–64.

14 Tektonidou MG: Renal involvement in the antiphospholipid syndrome (APS)-APS nephropathy. Clin Rev Allergy Immunol 2009; 36:131–140.

15 Bemanian S, Motallebi M, Nosrati SM: Cocaine-induced renal infarction: report of a case and review of the literature. BMC Nephrol 2005;6:10.

16 Frost L, Engholm G, Johnsen S, Møller H, Henneberg EW, Husted S: Incident thromboembolism in the aorta and the renal, mesenteric, pelvic, and extremity arteries after discharge from the hospital with a diagnosis of atrial fibrillation. Arch Intern Med 2001;161: 272–276.

17 Antopolsky M, Simanovsky N, Stalnikowicz R, Salameh S, Hiller N: Renal infarction in the ED: 10-year experience and review of the literature. Am J Emerg Med 2012;30:1055–1060.

18 Morris D, Kisly A, Stoyka CG, Provenzano R: Spontaneous bilateral renal artery occlusion associated with chronic atrial fibrillation. Clin Nephrol 1993;39:257–259.

19 Amilineni V, Lackner DF, Morse WS, Srinivas N: Contrast-enhanced CT for acute flank pain caused by acute renal artery occlusion. AJR Am J Roentgenol 2000;174:105–106.

20 Correas JM, Claudon M, Tranquart F, Hélénon O: [Contrast-enhanced ultrasonography: renal applications]. J Radiol 2003;84(12 pt 2):2041–2054.

21 Miyoshi T, Okayama H, Hiasa G, Kawata Y, Yamada T, Kazatani Y: Contrast-enhanced ultrasound for the evaluation of acute renal infarction. J Med Ultrason 2016;43:141–143.

22 Brandão LR, Simpson EA, Lau KK: Neonatal renal vein thrombosis. Semin Fetal Neonatal Med 2011;16:323–328.
23 Ogunbiyi OA: Renal vein thrombosis in patients with nephrotic syndrome: CT diagnosis. Afr J Med Med Sci 1995;24:33–40.
24 Biassoli E, Petrucci I, Meola M: Ruolo del color-Doppler nella diagnosi di trombosi primitiva della vena renale; in Aggiornamenti di Ecografia e Color Doppler, 2005, pp 115–119.
25 Petrucci I, Biassoli E, Frangioni S, Meola M: La trombosi secondaria della vena renale: casi clinici e revisione della letteratura; in Aggiornamenti di Ecografia e Color Doppler, 2005, pp 120–124.

Claudio Ronco, MD
Department of Nephrology Dialysis and Transplantation
International Renal Research Institute (IRRIV), San Bortolo Hospital
Viale Rodolfi 37, IT–36100 Vicenza (Italy)
E-Mail cronco@goldnet.it

Meola M, Petrucci I, Ronco C (eds): Ultrasound Imaging in Acute and Chronic Kidney Disease.
Contrib Nephrol. Basel, Karger, 2016, vol 188, pp 64–68 (DOI: 10.1159/000445468)

Clinical Scenarios in Acute Kidney Injury: Post-Renal Acute Kidney Injury

Mario Meola[a, b] · Sara Samoni[a, c] · Ilaria Petrucci[a, b] · Claudio Ronco[c]

[a]Sant'Anna School of Advanced Studies, Pisa, [b]Department of Internal Medicine, University of Pisa, Pisa, and [c]Department of Nephrology Dialysis and Transplantation, International Renal Research Institute (IRRIV), San Bortolo Hospital, Vicenza, Italy

Abstract

The incidence of acute kidney injury related to urinary tract obstruction is low (1–10%). It occurs in bilateral renal or lower urinary tract obstruction or in ureter obstruction in patients with a single functioning kidney or with pre-existing chronic kidney disease. The etiology and the incidence of obstruction vary on the basis of age and gender. Conventional ultrasound has a high sensitivity (>95%), but low specificity (<70%) in the diagnosis of urinary tract obstruction. Nevertheless, color Doppler is used through the evaluation of renal resistive indexes, ureteral jet and twinkling artifact.

Incidence and Etiology of Post-Renal AKI

The incidence of acute kidney injury (AKI) related to urinary tract obstruction ranges between 1 and 10% of AKI [1]. Among these cases, <5% requires surgical intervention [2]. A single functioning kidney can maintain the normal excretory function as well as the hydrosaline and acid–base balance, and this explains the low incidence of post-renal AKI. Subsequently, post-renal AKI occurs only in bilateral renal or lower urinary tract obstruction (bladder neck, urethra) (fig. 1) or in ureter obstruction in patients with a single functioning kidney (fig. 2) or with pre-existing chronic kidney disease.

The etiology and the incidence of obstruction vary on the basis of age and gender (table 1). During childhood, the most common causes of post-renal AKI are congenital stenosis (urethra, uretero-pelvic junction, uretero-vesical

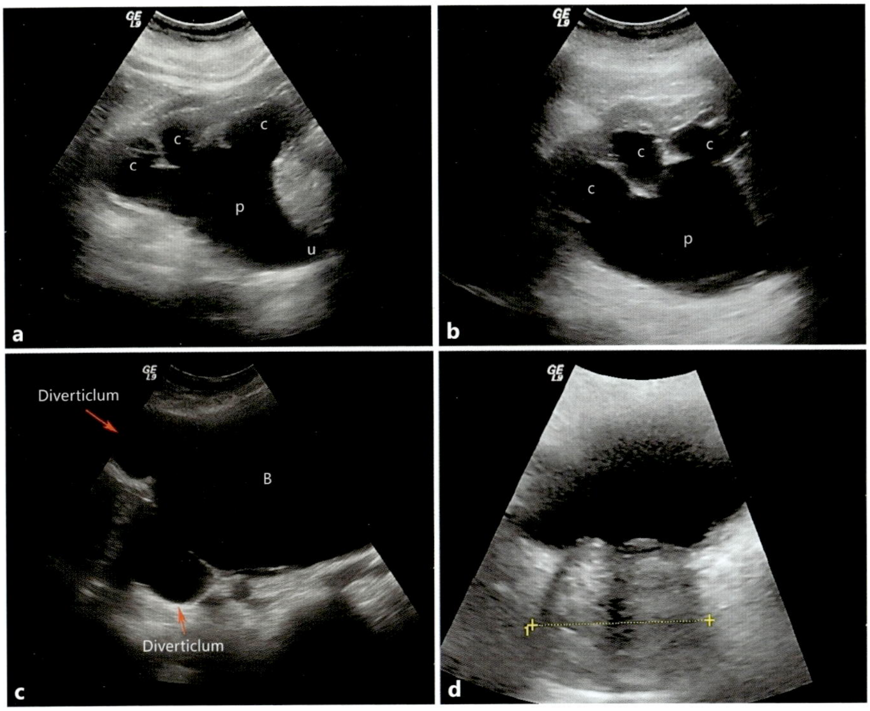

Fig. 1. AKI due to acute urinary tract obstruction in a patient with benign prostatic hypertrophy. The patient had worsening renal function (serum creatinine 4.8 mg/dl) and anuria. **a**, **b** Massive bilateral hydronephrosis: renal calyces of both sides were dilated, corticalized and with rounded contours. Renal pelvis and ureters were ectatic, without malformation. **c** Bladder had multiple parietal diverticula. **d** Benign prostatic hypertrophy: Transversal diameter 63 mm. c = Calyces; p = pelvis; u = ureter; B = bladder.

junction), vesico-ureteral reflux and urolithiasis. In young and adult men, the most common cause of temporary urinary obstruction is kidney stones, while in young women it is more frequently related to gynecological surgery, pregnancy or pelvic organs cancer. In patients >60 years, urinary obstruction is more frequent in men than in women and it is commonly due to prostate hypertrophy or, occasionally, prostate cancer with infiltration of seminal vesicles and ureteral orifice.

Imaging in Clinical Work-Up of Post-Renal AKI

Conventional ultrasound (US) has a key role in the diagnosis of urinary obstruction [3]. Despite its high sensitivity (>95%), the detection of a urinary tract dilation does not necessarily mean the presence of an obstruction [4], thus

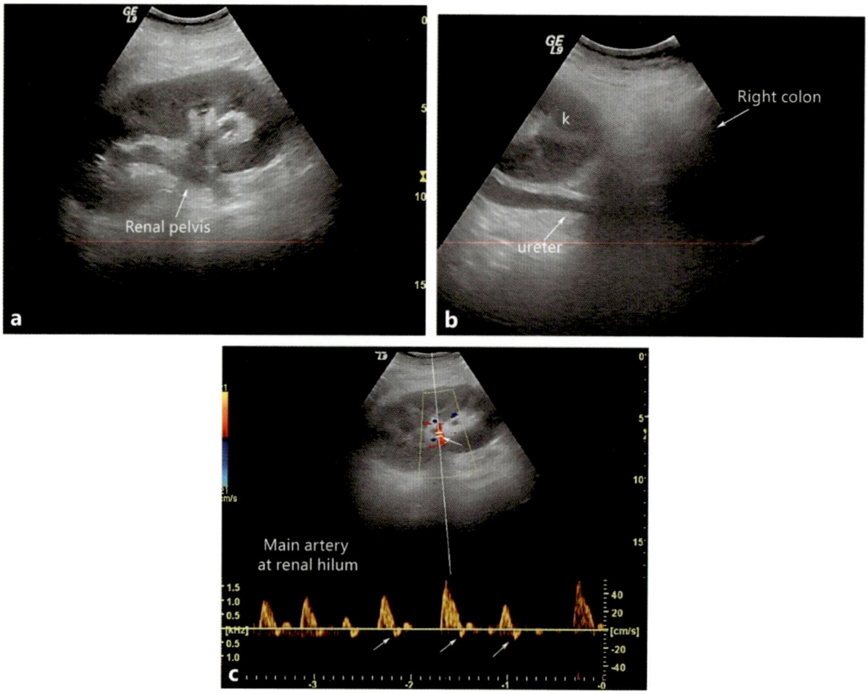

Fig. 2. AKI due to acute urinary tract obstruction in single kidney patient. A 78-year-old male with severe systemic arteriopathy (previous acute myocardial infarction, aortocoronary bypass, aorto-bi iliac graft, obliterative arterial disease of the lower limbs, previous transient ischemic attacks), atrial fibrillation, previous left nephrectomy due to neoplasm and recent acute right renal artery thrombosis treated with fibrinolysis. His baseline serum creatinine (sCr) was 1.8 mg/dl. Three months after the acute right renal artery thrombosis, he spontaneously stopped the anticoagulant therapy and had a worsening of renal function (sCr 9.8 mg/dl) with renal colic and anuria. Laboratory examinations showed leukocytosis, while LDH was 187 UI/l. **a** Right kidney was enlarged (coronal diameter 13.5 cm), hypoechoic and without vascularization. **b** Upper urinary tract was dilated until medium ureter. Renal artery was patent. **c** At renal hilum, vascular signal was arrhythmic, characterized by high peripheral resistances (not only with marked differences between peak systolic velocities and end-diastolic velocities, but also with reverse flow). Abdomen X-rays did not show radiopaque stones. Spiral CT displayed a juxta-vesical ureteral lithiasis (4–5 mm). The urinary tract obstruction was treated by ureteroscopy and double-J stenting. Patient was discharged with sCr 2.1 mg/dl. k = Kidney.

reducing its specificity (<70%) [5]. When the virtual excretory system is dilated by urine stagnation, an anechoic, multi-loculated, fluid collection appears into the hyperechoic renal sinus. The fluid collection highlights the upper urinary tract. Renal calyces appear as multiple small anechoic circular gaps, which are closely linked with renal parenchyma and communicate with each other. They flow together into a large central gap characterized by a triangular or rounded

Table 1. Post-renal AKI etiology

Acute bilateral ureter obstruction or unilateral ureter obstruction in single kidney
Intrinsic obstruction (lithiasis, clots, papillary necrosis, uric acid crystals, hyphae, post-surgical edema)
Extraluminal obstruction (ureter surgical ligature)
Paraluminal obstruction (fibrosis, retroperitoneal effusion)
Low urinary tract obstruction (bladder neck)
Intrinsic obstruction (lithiasis, clots, papillary necrosis, vesical neoplasm, urinary tract infections with edema, neurologic bladder, anti-depressive drugs)
Extraluminal obstruction (benign prostate hypertrophy, prostate cancer)
Urethral obstruction (commonly chronic)
Phimosis, congenital valves, urethral stenosis, neoplasms

shape (pelvis). The renal pelvis converges into the ureter, a small duct with a variable diameter on the basis of hydronephrosis severity. Ureter runs along the medial profile of psoas muscle, crosses the external iliac vessels and arrives into the small pelvis.

There are several physiological and para-physiological conditions that may lead to a slight hypotonia of the excretory system (hyperhydration, diuretics use, pregnancy, mega-calycosis). These circumstances, as well as some anatomical abnormalities, such as extra-renal pelvis and para-pelvic cysts, must be taken into account in the differential diagnosis [3]. Conversely, pathological conditions, such as retroperitoneal fibrosis, post-actinic ureteral lesions and lymphomatous infiltration may cause ureteral obstruction without evident urinary tract dilation.

The major limits of US in the diagnosis and the follow-up of hydronephrosis are its low specificity and the poor visibility of lumbar and pelvic ureter. As mentioned above, the occurrence of urinary tract dilation does not necessarily mean the presence of an obstruction. The low specificity of US could partially be overcome by means of color Doppler through the visualization of ureteral jet and the measurement of renal resistive indexes. In fact, the presence of ureteral jet, related to urine excretion into the bladder, could assess function and patency of the ureter [6]. Regarding renal hemodynamic in urinary tract obstruction, it has been shown that RIs are significantly higher in obstructed than in non-obstructed kidneys [7]. However, an intermittent or partial hydronephrosis that alters renal hemodynamics may lead to a wrong diagnosis.

The sensitivity of Doppler is reduced in cases of hyperhydration, administration of non-steroidal anti-inflammatory drugs or diuretics. The stimulated diuresis test [8], the evaluation of ureteral jet and of twinkling artifact could be useful for the differential diagnosis [6]. Twinkling artifact is a color Doppler phenomenon that may facilitate the detection of nephrolithiasis. This artifact is commonly observed at color Doppler imaging when rough reflective surfaces, such as renal calculi, are insonated. It appears as a comet tail behind the hyperechoic line produced by calculi with alternating colors [9].

Conclusion

Conventional US has a high sensitivity in the diagnosis and in the follow-up of urinary obstruction. Moreover, its low specificity could be overcome by means of color Doppler through the evaluation of RI, ureteral jet and twinkling artifact.

References

1 Liaño F, Pascual J: Epidemiology of acute renal failure: a prospective, multicenter, community-based study. Madrid acute renal failure study group. Kidney Int 1996;50:811–818.
2 Licurse A, Kim MC, Dziura J, Forman HP, Formica RN, Makarov DV, Parikh CR, Gross CP: Renal ultrasonography in the evaluation of acute kidney injury: developing a risk stratification framework. Arch Intern Med 2010;170:1900–1907.
3 Webb JA: Regular review ultrasonography in the diagnosis of renal obstruction. BMJ 1990;301:944–946.
4 Rascoff JH, Golden RA, Spinowitz BS, Charytan C: Nondilated obstructive nephropathy. Arch Intern Med 1983;143:696–698.
5 Ellenbogen PH, Scheible FW, Talner LB, Leopold GR: Sensitivity of gray scale ultrasound in detecting urinary tract obstruction. AJR Am J Roentgenol 1978;130:731–733.
6 Bertolotto M, Perrone R, Rimondini A: [Kidney obstruction: potential use of ultrasonography and Doppler color ultrasonography]. Arch Ital Urol Androl 2000;72:127–134.
7 Pepe P, Motta L, Pennisi M, Aragona F: Functional evaluation of the urinary tract by color-Doppler ultrasonography (CDU) in 100 patients with renal colic. Eur J Radiol 2005;53:131–135.
8 Meola M, Giuliano G, Morelli E, Cupisti A, Barsotti G: Ultrasound diagnosis of suspected urinary tract obstruction using a stimulated diuresis test. Nephron 1995;71:143–148.
9 Dillman JR, Kappil M, Weadock WJ, Rubin JM, Platt JF, DiPietro MA, Bude RO: Sonographic twinkling artifact for renal calculus detection: correlation with CT. Radiology 2011;259:911–916.

Claudio Ronco, MD
Director of Department of Nephrology Dialysis and Transplantation
International, Renal Research Institute (IRRIV), San Bortolo Hospital
Viale Roldolfi 37, IT–36100 Vicenza (Italy)
E-Mail cronco@goldnet.it

Meola M, Petrucci I, Ronco C (eds): Ultrasound Imaging in Acute and Chronic Kidney Disease.
Contrib Nephrol. Basel, Karger, 2016, vol 188, pp 69–80 (DOI: 10.1159/000445469)

Imaging in Chronic Kidney Disease

Mario Meola[a, b] • Sara Samoni[a, c] • Ilaria Petrucci[a, b]

[a]Sant'Anna School of Advanced Studies, Pisa, [b]Department of Internal Medicine, University of Pisa, Pisa, and [c]Department of Nephrology Dialysis and Transplantation, International Renal Research Institute (IRRIV), San Bortolo Hospital, Vicenza, Italy

Abstract

Chronic kidney disease (CKD) diagnosis and staging are based on estimated or calculated glomerular filtration rate (GFR), urinalysis and kidney structure at renal imaging techniques. Ultrasound (US) has a key role in evaluating both morphological changes (by means of B-Mode) and patterns of vascularization (by means of color-Doppler and contrast-enhanced US), thus contributing to CKD diagnosis and to the follow-up of its progression. In CKD, conventional US allows measuring longitudinal diameter and cortical thickness and evaluating renal echogenicity and urinary tract status. Maximum renal length is usually considered a morphological marker of CKD, as it decreases contemporarily to GFR, and should be systematically recorded in US reports. More recently, it has been found to be a significant correlation of both renal longitudinal diameter and cortical thickness with renal function. Conventional US should be integrated by color Doppler, which shows parenchymal perfusion and patency of veins and arteries, and by spectral Doppler, which is crucial for the diagnosis of renal artery stenosis and provides important information about intrarenal microcirculation. Different values of renal resistive indexes (RIs) have been associated with different primary diseases, as they reflect vascular compliance. Since RIs significantly correlate with renal function, they have been proposed to be independent risk factors for CKD progression, besides proteinuria, low GFR and arterial hypertension. Despite several new applications, US and color Doppler contribute to a definite diagnosis in <50% of cases of CKD, because of the lack of specific US patterns, especially in cases of advanced CKD. However, US is useful to evaluate CKD progression and to screen patients at risk for CKD. The indications and the recommended frequency of color Doppler US could differ in each case and the follow-up should be tailored.

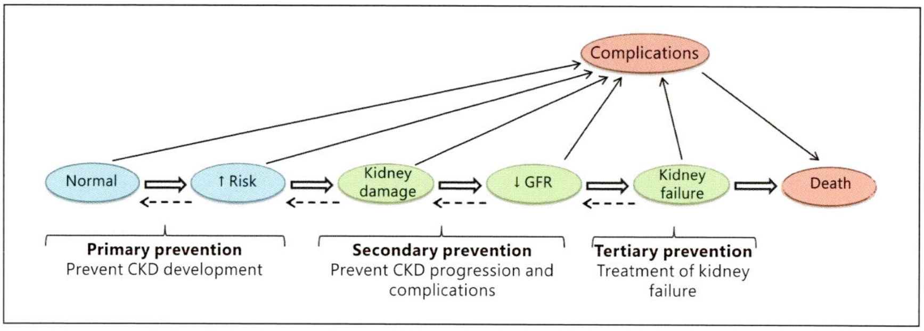

Fig. 1. Conceptual model of CKD. Algorithm represents the CKD progression, from the development to the occurrence of complications. Green circles symbolize CKD stage 3–5, blue circles preclinical phases (CKD stages 1–2 and increased risk for CKD), while pink circles the major outcomes such as end-stage renal disease and death. Thin arrows indicate risk factors related to the development and the progression of CKD. Empty arrows symbolize the potential reversibility of clinical phases. Complications represent the clinical manifestations due to CKD and its treatment as well as the consequences of the reduction of GFR and cardiovascular diseases associated to CKD. The objectives of primary, secondary and tertiary CKD prevention are to slow CKD progression, treat complications of CKD and reduce cardiovascular risk, thus improving patients' life quality and survival. Modified from National Kidney Foundation guidelines [2].

Definition, Staging and Progression of Chronic Kidney Disease

The National Kidney Foundation's Kidney Disease Quality Outcome Initiative (NKF-KDOQI) [1] has proposed the current conceptual model of chronic kidney disease (CKD) for the first time in 2002. Subsequently, this model was improved by the Kidney Disease: Improving Global Outcomes work group and, at last, approved in an international consensus conference in 2005 [2]. The conceptual model of CKD, showed in figure 1, contributed to improve definition, staging, prognosis, treatment and complications of CKD, as well as risk factors for CKD progression. The objective of this model was to develop programs for primary CKD prevention and improve outcomes in advanced stages of CKD (secondary and tertiary CKD prevention). Despite current clinical management of nephropathic patients including several strategies to slow CKD progression, reduce cardiovascular risk and treat CKD complications, thus improving patients' life quality and survival, there are still unsolved problems, such as the assessment of the impact of CKD on cardiovascular risk, the high frequency of late referral of nephropathic patients to nephrologists, the evaluation of the precise relationship between acute kidney injury (AKI) and CKD and the potential reversibility of CKD. Moreover, the definition of a normal range of values for glomerular filtration rate (GFR) in

Table 1. Stages of CKD

Stage	Description	GFR, ml/min/1.73 m^2
1	Kidney damage with normal or ↑ GFR	≥90
2	Kidney damage with mild ↓ GFR	60–89
3	Moderate ↓ GFR	30–59
4	Severe ↓ GFR	15–29
5	Kidney failure	<15 (or dialysis)

CKD is defined as either kidney damage or GFR <60 ml/min/1.73 m^2 for ≥3 months. Kidney damage is defined as pathologic abnormalities or markers of damage, including abnormalities in blood or urine tests or imaging studies.

the elderly is still controversial, as well as the clinical meaning of albuminuria in CKD patients. A multidisciplinary approach, including the analysis of epidemiological data, basic research and clinical investigations, may assess the efficacy of each therapeutic strategy and its ability to decrease the social burden of CKD.

CKD is diagnosed by the presence of either kidney damage or decreased kidney function (decreased GFR) for ≥3 months [1–3]. This definition provides objective diagnostic criteria, which can be easily checked by means of blood or urine samples or renal imaging.

The Cockcroft–Gault and the Modified Diet in Renal Disease equations are the most used formulas to estimate, respectively, creatinine clearance (CrCl) and GFR. They are both precise if GFR is less than 60 ml/min/1.73 m^2, while they lose accuracy in the presence of higher GRF values. In clinical settings where renal function must be precisely assessed, such as in potential kidney donors, 24-hour CrCl measurement is mandatory. However, in most cases, estimated GFR (eGFR) allows diagnosis, classification and evaluation of CKD progression [1, 3]. The CKD classification in 5 stages, based on the progressively worsening of GFR, is shown in table 1.

The aims of each therapeutic strategy used in CKD are to prevent the loss of renal function, to manage potential complications and to reduce cardiovascular risk.

The loss of renal function in CKD may widely vary. The rapid progression of CKD is defined as the decrease of GFR >4 ml/min/1.73 m^2/year. When it occurs, CKD stage 3 (GFR <60 ml/min/1.73 m^2) takes about 10 years to evolve in CKD stage 5 (15 ml/min/1.73 m^2). The progression of CKD occurs more rapidly in patients suffering from poorly controlled arterial hypertension, proteinuria and diabetes [4], while it slows by the administration of renin–angiotensin system inhibitors, which reduces both blood pressure and proteinuria.

The most common complications of CKD are arterial hypertension, anemia, malnutrition, mineral bone diseases, neuropathy and worsening of life quality. These complications mainly occur during CKD stage 4 and 5 (GFR <30 ml/min/1.73 m^2), but they may be prevented by early treatments. Moreover, it must be highlighted that CKD patients have a higher susceptibility to AKI related to surgical or medical potentially invasive procedures or exposure to toxic drugs than general population.

The presence of CKD is an independent risk factor for cardiovascular disease [5]. In CKD patients, cardiovascular events occur more frequently; treatment and prevention of cardiovascular diseases may both improve primary outcomes and reduce CKD progression, thus revealing a close linkage between heart and kidney [5, 6].

Prevalence and Etiology of CKD

CKD is a major cost driver for healthcare systems in developed countries. In fact, the number of patients with CKD is increasing due to the rise in the average population age and, subsequently, in the prevalence of age-related diseases, such as arterial hypertension and diabetes, that participate to the pathogenesis of CKD. Otherwise, CKD patients have 3- to 4-fold increased risk for cardiovascular mortality and 20- to 50-fold increased risk for dialysis, which is an expensive chronic treatment, compared to general population. It has been calculated that 363 patients per million population (pmp) started dialysis in 2013 in the United States [7].

Table 2 shows the classification of CKD on the basis of etiology proposed by NKF-KDOQI [1] and the prevalence of each etiology in patients with advanced CKD in United States, as reported in the United States Renal Data System [7]. It has been estimated that diabetes and arterial hypertension are the main causes for new entries in dialysis (72.5% of cases), while glomerular diseases represent the third cause (7.5%) followed by cystic diseases. Due to the high rate of late nephrology referral in CKD, 17.7% of new entries in dialysis are unknown or related to less frequent causes, such as hereditary kidney diseases, congenital abnormalities, vesico-ureteral reflux, chronic pyelonephritis and chronic interstitial nephropathy. In developed countries, the incidence of post-infective glomerulonephritis is decreasing, while nephropathy due to systemic diseases and chronic interstitial nephritis are becoming more frequent. Moreover, while hereditary and congenital diseases, glomerulonephritis and interstitial nephropathy are more frequent in adults, vascular and diabetic nephropathy outnumber in the elderly. The age-related

Table 2. Classification of CKD on the basis of pathophysiology [1], etiology [1] and prevalence (according to the USRDS) [7]

Pathophysiology	Etiology	Prevalence, %
Diabetic Glomerulosclerosis	Diabetes mellitus (type 1 and 2)	44
Primary or secondary glomerular diseases		7.5
Proliferative GN	SLE	
Membranoproliferative GN	Vasculitis	
Focal proliferative GN	Infective endocarditis	
Diffuse proliferative GN	Hepatitis B, C	
Crescentic GN	HIV	
Non-inflammatory glomerular diseases		
Minimal change disease		
Focal glomerulosclerosis		
Membranous GN		
Fibrillary GN		
Alport syndrome		
Vascular diseases		29
Large vessel diseases	Renal artery stenosis	
Medium vessel diseases	Arterial hypertension	
Nephrosclerosis		
Small vessel diseases	Sickle cell anemia	
Microangiopathy	HUS (including cyclosporine and tacrolimus toxicity)	
Tubulointerstitial diseases		4
Tubulointerstitial nephritis	Infection, lithiasis	
Pyelonephritis	NSAIDs	
Analgesic nephropathy	Antibiotics	
Interstitial allergic nephritis	Sarcoidosis	
Granulomatous interstitial nephritis	Uveitis	
Noninflammatory tubulointerstitial nephritis	Vesico-ureteral reflux	
Reflux nephropathy	Neoplasm, prostatism, lithiasis	
Obstructive nephropathy	Multiple myeloma	
Myelomatous kidney		
Cystic diseases		2
Polycystic disease	Autosomal dominant or recessive disorders	
Tuberous sclerosis		
Von Hippel Lindau syndrome		
Medullary cystic disease		
Kidney transplant		13.5
Chronic renal allograft rejection		
Drug toxicity	Cyclosporine/tacrolimus	
Recurrent disease	Glomerular diseases	
Transplant nephropathy		

USRDS = United States Renal Data System; GN = glomerulonephritis; SLE = systemic lupus erythematosus; HIV = human immunodeficiency virus; HUS = hemolytic uremic syndrome; NSAIDs = non-steroidal anti-inflammatory drugs.

diseases, such as atherosclerosis, diabetes and arterial hypertension, lead more frequently to a CKD characterized by the combination of different risk factors.

Imaging in Clinical Work-Up of CKD

CKD diagnosis and staging are based on estimated or calculated GFR, urinalysis (i.e., proteinuria, hematuria, hyposthenuria, etc.) and kidney structural abnormalities displayed by renal imaging techniques. Ultrasound (US) is usually the first medical test prescribed in subjects at risk for kidney damage as well as in nephropathic patients. Since renal biopsy and contrast media are contraindicated in CKD patients, US is crucial to evaluate both morphological changes (by means of B-Mode) and patterns of vascularization (by means of color Doppler and contrast-enhanced US [CEUS]), thus contributing to the diagnosis of CKD and its etiology.

At present, the use of CT and MRI in CKD patients is limited to the investigation of obstructive diseases, urinary tract abnormalities and renal artery diseases. The role of urography with intravenous contrast media is also restricted, since most of its indications are replaced by spiral CT. Nevertheless, renal scintigraphy is still used, especially in cases of monolateral renal diseases, to examine perfusion, function and excretion of each kidney, separately.

A protocol to prevent AKI related to contrast media (CI-AKI) should be used in cases in which a contrast-enhanced CT is mandatory. In fact, it has been estimated that CI-AKI occurs in approximately 6% of patients who underwent contrast-enhanced CT, and in 1% of cases, CI-AKI evolves in CKD [8]. Moreover, as we mentioned above, CKD patients have a higher susceptibility to CI-AKI. Similarly, MRI with gadolinium chelate is also contraindicated in CKD patients for the risk of nephrogenic systemic fibrosis (NSF). In the future, the development of CEUS may become critical in CKD patients.

In CKD, conventional US allows to measure longitudinal diameter and cortical thickness and to evaluate renal echogenicity and urinary tract (fig. 2). Renal longitudinal diameter is usually taken into account as a morphological marker of CKD, as it decreases contemporarily to GFR. In fact, despite few old studies showing a high correlation of GFR and renal volume [9], the measurement of maximum renal length of both kidneys is recommended [10] and should be systematically recorded in ultrasonography reports. In a more recent study performed in the elderly renal volume and longitudinal diameter correlates with GFR, although renal volume is more predictive to progression of CKD [11]. Currently, the calculation of renal volume by means of longitudinal,

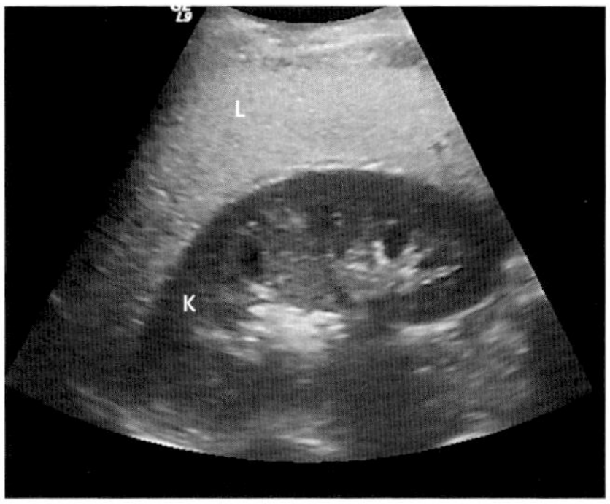

Fig. 2. Normal kidney. At B-mode examination, the echogenicity of the kidneys is compared to the one of liver and of spleen. In figure 2, the right normal kidney appears hypoechoic in comparison to the liver because of the presence of severe liver steatosis. K = Kidney; L = liver.

transversal and anteroposterior diameters is not always feasible and the use of ellipsoid formula is not appropriate because of the variability of renal shape [12]. Moreover, the low correlation between renal volume and GFR found in some studies [13] may be explained by the inclusion of renal sinus in the calculation of total renal volume. In fact, renal sinus does not contain parenchyma and it differs for dimension in general population as well as in CKD patients. In chronic interstitial nephropathy, an atrophic index has been proposed to assess the progression of CKD. It is calculated by dividing renal longitudinal diameter by sinus longitudinal diameter, both measured in the same coronal scan [14]. In addition, some authors found a better correlation between GFR and cortical thickness measured in sagittal scan as the distance of basis of mesorenal medullar pyramid from renal capsule [15, 16]. It may be explained by the progressive increase of cortical hyperechogenicity [17] and the decrease of cortical thickness [15] in CKD patients. Both variations also occur in cases characterized by a normal longitudinal diameter or in cases of sinus sclerolipomatosis. In a recent study performed in 176 patients with different stages of CKD, renal length and cortical thickness (especially left cortical thickness) were correlated with renal function [18].

Conventional kidney B-Mode US should be integrated by color Doppler, which provides semi-quantitative parameters such as parenchymal perfusion, presence or absence of blood flow, patency of veins and arteries (fig. 3). Despite the usefulness of color Doppler, it does not often allow definitive diagnosis. Spectral Doppler, by which velocity (v)/time (t) curves can be obtained in principal as well as in interlobar arteries, is crucial for diagnosis of several pathological conditions. In fact, the measurement of systolic peak velocity and end-diastolic velocity in renal arteries is sufficient to diagnose or exclude the presence of a renal artery stenosis. Calculation of renal resistive indexes (RIs) in interlobar arteries by means of spectral Doppler provides important information about intrarenal microvasculature. In CKD, the progressive decrease of

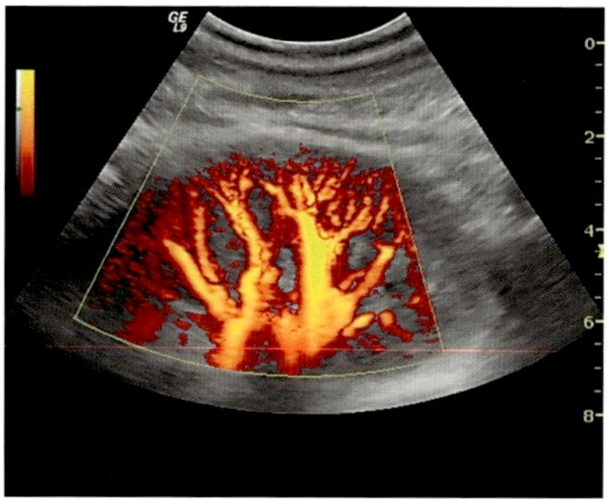

Fig. 3. Renal parenchymal blushing. The assessment of renal perfusion with color color Doppler technique is important but commonly does not guarantee a conclusive differential diagnosis.

functioning renal mass is accompanied by a parallel decrease of renal blood flow. This is represented in spectral Doppler with a decreased width of the v/t curve and a slower diastolic flow.

When the main damage is localized in the vessels wall, such as in cases of atherosclerotic remodeling, microcirculation thrombosis, atheroembolism and vasculitis, the capacitance (vascular compliance) and the total microvasculature cross-sectional area decrease (fig. 4). The increase in total vascular impedance leads to a marked pulsatile flow with a decreased diastolic perfusion and a subsequent RIs increase (>0.75). The RIs increase is related to arterial stiffness and increased hydraulic resistance [19] and it significantly correlates with atherosclerotic damage of renal microvasculature [20]. When the interstitial infiltration-fibrosis is predominant, the transmural pressure increases leading to a marked capacitance decrease. RIs are usually <0.75. Boddi et al. [21] demonstrated that RIs measurement allows an early identification of patients affected by chronic tubulointerstitial nephritis. In glomerulonephritis, the intrarenal vascular resistance increases to a lesser degree. As glomerulus sclerosis progressively develops, blood flow shunts from afferent to efferent arterioles, thus usually leading to RIs ≤0.70. A study on 86 CKD patients with an average follow-up of 5 years, showed a slower GFR decrease in patients with initial RIs ≤0.61 or 0.62–0.69 than in those with initial RIs ≥0.70. In 6-year follow-up, subjects with RIs ≥0.70 showed a decrease in GFR >50%, while in those with RIs <0.70, GFR decreases of 33% [22]. Therefore, RIs >0.70 are predictive for a faster progression of CKD, regardless of the initial GFR value. In advanced CKD, progressive glomerular sclerosis, tubular atrophy and interstitial fibrosis are common in all diseases. In these patients, RIs are >0.70 and reach values >0.80 in last phases, independently by primary kidney injury. RIs >80 are associated with poor and slow blood flow and few possibilities of renal recovery, as it is well-documented in the transplanted kidney [23] as well as in the native kidney after renal artery stenosis correction [24]. Since RIs significantly correlate with renal function,

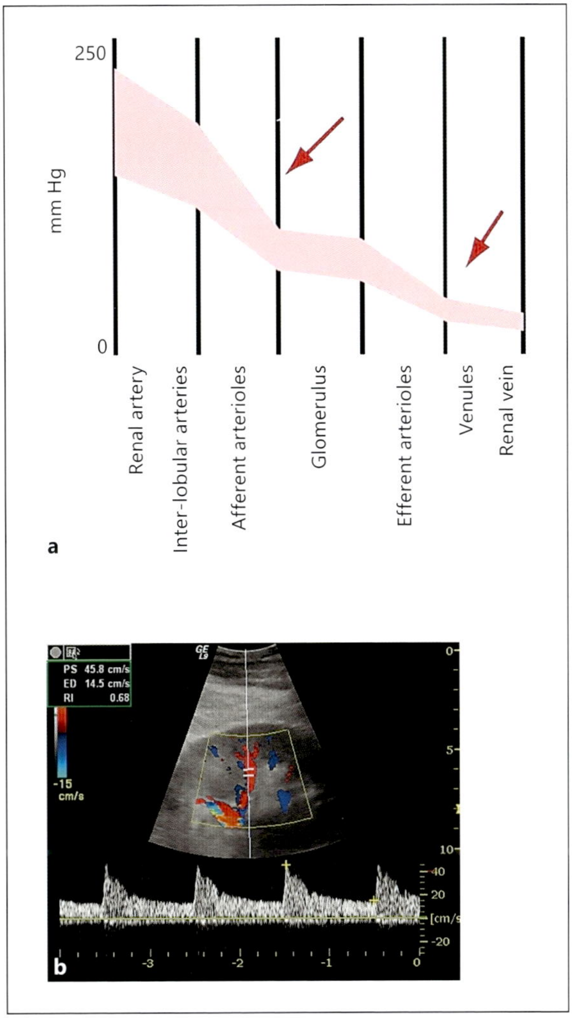

Fig. 4. Intra-parenchymal renal vascular resistance and renal RIs variation. **a** Diagram showing intrarenal resistances. Pre-glomerular microvessels are responsible for the main vascular resistances. **b** In healthy adults, RIs measured in inter-lobar arteries are <0.60. In patients affected by CKD, RIs depend on primary disease. In fact, when primary disease is interstitial, they are usually >0.70 while, in cases of glomerulonephritis, they are <0.70. When microvessels are largely affected by the disease, RIs are often >0.75. The presence of RIs >0.80 has a negative prognostic significance for renal recovery, in native and transplant kidneys.

they have been proposed as independent risk factors for the progression of CKD, besides proteinuria, low GFR and arterial hypertension [25].

Table 3 summarizes kidney abnormalities that could be detected by imaging techniques in CKD patients.

At present, a better assessment of kidney perfusion is possible thanks to CEUS technique, which allows evaluation of vessels with a diameter <400 μm. Nevertheless, the precise role of dynamic CEUS in the management of CKD is still undefined, except for chronic ischemic disease and atheroembolic nephropathy. Moreover, although the use of elastosonography in native kidneys seems to be restricted, further studies are needed to clarify its role in the assessment of CKD.

Table 3. Structural abnormalities of kidneys displayed by the main imaging techniques and potential related kidney diseases. Modified from National Kidney Foundation guidelines [2]

Imaging technique	Kidney diseases
US and color-Doppler	
General appearance	Nephrocalcinosis, hydronephrosis, cystic or solid lesions
Hyperechogenicity	Microcystic disease or medical nephropathy
Small hyperechoic kidneys	CKD
Nephromegaly	Neoplasms, infiltrative diseases, nephrotic syndrome, early stages of diabetes
Renal asymmetry/scars	Vascular or urological diseases, tubulointerstitial diseases due to infections/lithiasis
Doppler analysis	Renal artery stenosis, renal vein thrombosis
Urography	Morphological or functional renal asymmetry, obstructive lithiasis, neoplasms, scars, calyces/ureteral abnormalities
CT	Obstructions, neoplasms, cysts, lithiasis, renal artery stenosis, acute or chronic pyelonephritis
MRI	Solid or cystic lesions, renal vein thrombosis, renal artery stenosis
Nuclear medicine techniques	Morphological or functional renal asymmetry, renal artery stenosis, acute or chronic pyelonephritis

Conclusion

Despite several new applications, US and color Doppler contribute to a definite diagnosis in <50% of cases of CKD. Its poor sensitivity in diagnosis is due to the lack of specific ultrasonographic patterns, especially in cases of advanced CKD. However, US is useful to evaluate CKD progression and to screen patients at risk for CKD, such as subjects with kidney stones, recurring urinary infections, vesico-ureteral reflux, polycystic diseases or hydronephrosis related to intrinsic or extrinsic urinary tract obstruction or vesico-ureteral reflux. The indications and the recommended frequency of color Doppler US in CKD patients and in subjects at risk for CKD could differ in each case and the follow-up should be tailored.

References

1 Eknoyan G, Levin NW: K/DOQI clinical practice guidelines for chronic kidney disease: evaluation, classification, and stratification. Am J Kidney Dis 2002;39(2 suppl 1):S1–S266.

2 Levey AS, Eckardt KU, Tsukamoto Y, Levin A, Coresh J, Rossert J, De Zeeuw D, Hostetter TH, Lameire N, Eknoyan G: Definition and classification of chronic kidney disease: a position statement from kidney disease: improving global outcomes (KDIGO). Kidney Int 2005;67:2089–2100.

3 Levey AS, Coresh J, Balk E, Kausz AT, Levin A, Steffes MW, Hogg RJ, Perrone RD, Lau J, Eknoyan G: Clinical guidelines national kidney foundation practice guidelines for chronic kidney: evaluation, classification, and stratification. Ann Intern Med 2003;139:137–147.

4 Levey AS, Schoolwerth AC, Burrows NR, Williams DE, Stith KR, McClellan W: Comprehensive public health strategies for preventing the development, progression, and complications of CKD: report of an expert panel convened by the centers for disease control and prevention. Am J Kidney Dis 2009;53:522–535.

5 Go AS, Chertow GM, Fan D, Mcculloch CE, Hsu CY: Chronic kidney disease and the risks of death, cardiovascular events, and hospitalization. N Engl J Med 2004;351:1296–1305.

6 Di Lullo L, House A, Gorini A, Santoboni A, Russo D, Ronco C: Chronic kidney disease and cardiovascular complications. Heart Fail Rev 2015;20:259–272.

7 US Renal Data System: 2015 Annual Data Report. Volume 2: End-Stage Renal Disease in the United States.

8 Kooiman J, Pasha SM, Zondag W, Sijpkens YW, van der Molen AJ, Huisman MV, Dekkers OM: Meta-analysis: serum creatinine changes following contrast enhanced CT imaging. Eur J Radiol 2012;81:2554–2561.

9 Emamian SA, Nielsen MB, Pedersen JF, Ytte L: Kidney dimensions at sonography: correlation with age, sex, and habitus in 665 adult volunteers. AJR Am J Roentgenol 1993;160:83–86.

10 American College of Radiology (in collaboration with the American Institute of Ultrasound in Medicine AIUM): ACR practice guideline for the performance of an ultrasound examination of the abdomen and/or retro-peritoneum. http://www.acr.org/guidelines.

11 Van Den Noortgate N, Velghe A, Petrovic M, Vandewiele C, Lameire N, Voet D, Afschrift M: The role of ultrasonography in the assessment of renal function in the elderly. J Nephrol 2003;16:658–662.

12 Bakker J, Olree M, Kaatee R, de Lange EE, Moons KG, Beutler JJ, Beek FJ: Renal volume measurements: accuracy and repeatability of US compared with that of MR imaging. Radiology 1999;211:623–628.

13 Sanusi AA, Arogundade FA, Famurewa OC, Akintomide AO, Soyinka FO, Ojo OE, Akinsola A: Relationship of ultrasonographically determined kidney volume with measured GFR, calculated creatinine clearance and other parameters in chronic kidney disease (CKD). Nephrol Dial Transplant 2009;24:1690–1694.

14 Sugiura T, Nakamori A, Wada A, Fukuhara Y: Evaluation of tubulointerstitial injury by Doppler ultrasonography in glomerular diseases. Clin Nephrol 2004;61:119–126.

15 Moghazi S, Jones E, Schroepple J, Arya K, Mcclellan W, Hennigar RA, O'Neill WC: Correlation of renal histopathology with sonographic findings. Kidney Int 2005;67:1515–1520.

16 Beland MD, Walle NL, Machan JT, Cronan JJ: Renal cortical thickness measured at ultrasound: is it better than renal length as an indicator of renal function in chronic kidney disease? AJR Am J Roentgenol 2010;195:W146–W149.

17 Khati NJ, Hill MC, Kimmel PL: The role of ultrasound in renal insufficiency: the essentials. Ultrasound Q 2005;21:227–244.

18 Takata T, Koda M, Sugihara T, Sugihara S, Okamoto T, Miyoshi K, Hodotsuka M, Fujise Y, Matono T, Okano J, Hosho K, Iyama T, Fukui T, Fukuda S, Munemura C, Isomoto H: Left renal cortical thickness measured by ultrasound can predict early progression of chronic kidney disease. Nephron 2016;132:25–32.

19 Bude RO, Rubin JM: Experimental studies relationship between the resistive index and vascular compliance and resistance. Radiology 1999;211:411–417.
20 Calabia J, Torguet P, Garcia I, Martin N, Mate G, Marin A, Molina C, Valles M: The relationship between renal resistive index, arterial stiffness, and atherosclerotic burden: the link between macrocirculation and microcirculation. J Clin Hypertens (Greenwich) 2014;16:186–191.
21 Boddi M, Cecioni I, Poggesi L, Fiorentino F, Olianti K, Berardino S, La Cava G, Gensini G: Renal resistive index early detects chronic tubulointerstitial nephropathy in normo- and hypertensive patients. Am J Nephrol 2006;26: 16–21.
22 Parolini C, Noce A, Staffolani E, Giarrizzo GF, Costanzi S, Splendiani G: Renal resistive index and long-term outcome in chronic nephropathies. Radiology 2009;252:888–896.
23 Radermacher J, Mengel M, Ellis S, Stuht S, Hiss M, Schwarz A, Eisenberger U, Burg M, Luft FC, Gwinner W, Haller H: The renal arterial resistance index and renal allograft survival. N Engl J Med 2003;349:115–124.
24 Radermacher J, Chavan A, Bleck J, Vitzthum A, Stoess B, Gebel Mj, Galanski M, Koch Km, Haller H: Use of Doppler ultrasonography to predict the outcome of therapy for renal-artery stenosis. N Engl J Med 2001;344:410–417.
25 Sugiura T, Wada A: Resistive index predicts renal prognosis in chronic kidney disease: results of a 4-year follow-up. Clin Exp Nephrol 2011;15:114–120.

Mario Meola, MD, PhD
Department of Internal Medicine
Sant'Anna School of Advanced Studies, University of Pisa
Via Savi 10, IT–56126 Pisa (Italy)
E-Mail mario.meola@unipi.it; m.meola@sssup.it

Meola M, Petrucci I, Ronco C (eds): Ultrasound Imaging in Acute and Chronic Kidney Disease.
Contrib Nephrol. Basel, Karger, 2016, vol 188, pp 81–88 (DOI: 10.1159/000445470)

Clinical Scenarios in Chronic Kidney Disease: Vascular Chronic Diseases

Mario Meola[a, b] · Sara Samoni[a, c] · Ilaria Petrucci[a, b]

[a]Sant'Anna School of Advanced Studies, Pisa, [b]Department of Internal Medicine, University of Pisa, Pisa, and [c]Department of Nephrology Dialysis and Transplantation, International Renal Research Institute (IRRIV), San Bortolo Hospital, Vicenza, Italy

Abstract

Vascular chronic diseases represent one of the leading causes of end-stage renal disease in incident dialysis patients. B-Mode ultrasound (US) and color Doppler (CD) have a high sensitivity and specificity in the diagnosis of vascular chronic diseases. US and CD should be used to identify subjects in the high risk population who are affected by main renal artery stenosis (RAS) and to identify and characterize patients without RAS who have chronic ischemic nephropathy caused by nephroangiosclerosis and/or atheroembolic disease. The most important CD parameters in the work-up of suspected RAS are increased peak systolic velocity and diastolic velocity, spectral broadening, high renal:aortic ratio and lateralization of renal resistive indexes (RIs). In the absence of direct or indirect signs of RAS, increases in intraparenchymal RIs, associated with systemic atherosclerotic disease, are indicative of microcirculation damage related to nephroangiosclerosis or atheroembolic disease.

Main Renal Artery Diseases

B-Mode ultrasound (US) does not have a pivotal role in differential diagnosis of renovascular disease but may show non-specific signs such as renal asymmetry, parenchymal thinning, flattening of the mesorenal column, aortic atheromatous disease or aneurysms and/or abnormalities of the renal artery course. Diagnosis of renal artery stenosis (RAS) is based only on a significant increase of systolic-diastolic velocity and a broadening of the velocity spectrum into the stenotic segment (fig. 1).

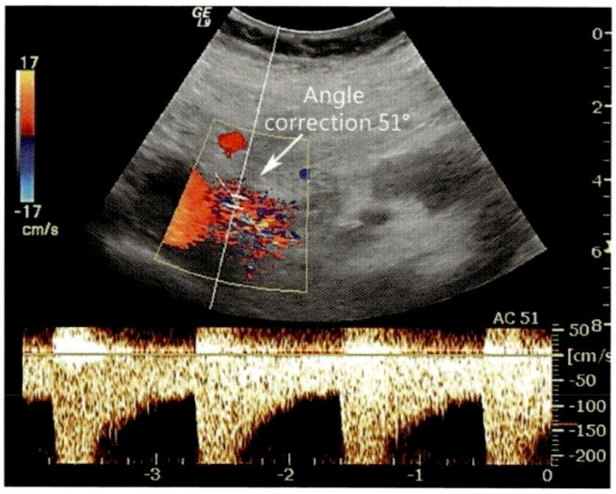

Fig. 1. Ostial RAS. Axial oblique scan of the left renal artery at the hilum. All signs of critical stenosis are present: aliasing and vascular bruit at color Doppler; systo-diastolic acceleration (peak systolic velocity >200 cm/s and diastolic velocity >90 cm/s), spectral broadening and wall thump at spectral sampling.

Blood flow is accelerated in the stenotic segment due to an increased trans-stenotic pressure gradient in order to maintain the continuity of downstream flow. Blood velocity increases (Venturi's effect) until a critical limit beyond which the trans-stenotic gradient is no longer able to overcome the stenosis' resistance. In this phase, the downstream flow rate is reduced while vortices and random flow lines movements disperse the pressure energy into heat. In pre-occlusive stenosis, spectral curve is characterized by an important decrease of the systo-diastolic gap with an almost complete disappearance of the diastolic component. In renal artery obstruction, orthodromic flow disappears and color Doppler (CD) shows only weak systolic ejection cones. Ischemic kidney structure varies depending on the clinical context in which the diagnosis is made. In early stages, when hemodynamic disturbances prevail (renovascular hypertension, reduction of the glomerular filtration rate), kidney size appears normal or slightly reduced. If RAS remains misdiagnosed, ischemia causes a progressive loss of nephronic mass (1 cm of longitudinal diameter/year). Factors that determine kidney damage are not yet well known, as atherosclerotic stenosis is commonly overlapped with an important damage of the microcirculation (caused by nephrosclerosis or, rarely, by atheroembolism; fig. 2).

Current pathophysiological interpretation is that stenosis synergistically acts with other progression factors (adaptive response of the renin-angiotensin system, dyslipidemia, atherogenic factors, hypoxia and oxidative stress) causing glomerulosclerosis, interstitial and vascular fibrosis. Indeed, glomeruli are affected only in end stages, while the prevalent injury would be interstitial fibrosis and progressive reduction of the cortical microcirculation [1].

These findings could justify the results of ASTRAL [2] and CORAL [3] studies, which have documented the inefficacy of revascularization on primary stenosis outcomes (kidney function and high blood pressure) if compared with medical therapy. Interstitial damage causes a progressive volume reduction and ischemic kidney becomes asymmetric and smaller than the contralateral.

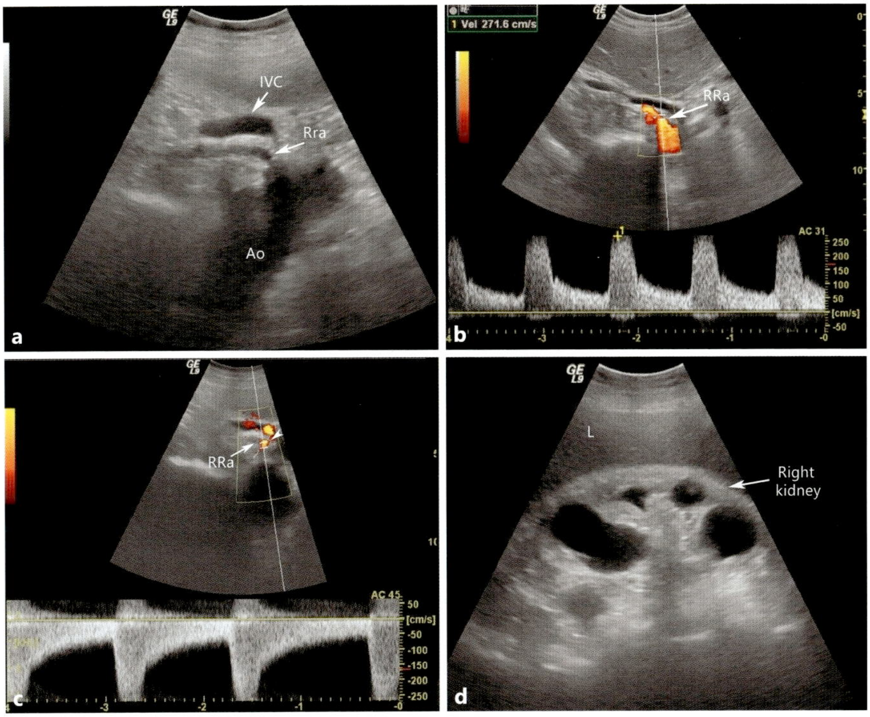

Fig. 2. Chronic ischemic nephropathy. Male, aged 78 years, with a history of ischemic heart disease and hypertension. In 2008, US revealed right kidney volume reduction (serum creatinine [sCr] 3.3 mg/dl, creatinine clearance [CrCL] 22 ml/min) with an aortic aneurysm and an atherosclerotic plaque extended to the ostium of both renal arteries. Three years after the first observation, sCr was 5 mg/dl, CrCL was 11 ml/min and proteinuria <1 g/day with refractory hypertension. **a** Origin of the right renal artery with mixed atheromasia. **b** Slow ostial cone ejection, without critical accelerations. Spectral width was reduced and diastolic flow was absent. **c** At 1 cm from the origin, a collateral vessel showed an important acceleration >250 cm/s. **d** The right kidney appeared hyperechoic with several acquired cysts and a little parenchymal polar residual portion where RIs were lateralized if compared to the contralateral kidney (0.56 vs 0.78). Ao = Aorta; Rra and RRa = right renal artery; IVC = inferior vena cava; L = liver.

Morphology of the ischemic kidney depends on the time of diagnosis. Thus, if the kidney maintains a normal volume, parenchyma appears thinned and hypoechoic. In advanced nephropathy, RAS is not assessable with CD due to the complete loss of flow and kidney's morphology being similar to that of other forms of CKD. Resistive indexes (RIs) behavior, calculated into the mesorenal interlobar arteries, reproduces the hemodynamic stages of the disease. If RAS is the prevalent damage, hypoperfusion causes a fall of renal flow and RIs, due to the activation of autoregulation mechanisms. RIs values in the ischemic kidney are much lower compared to the contralateral kidney ($\Delta > 0.12$), where vascular

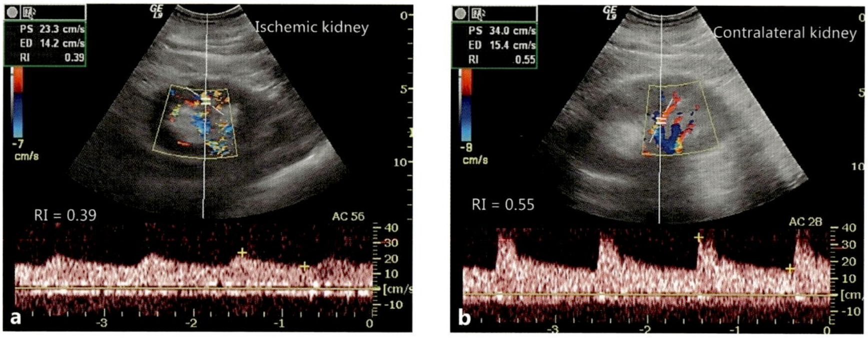

Fig. 3. Lateralization of intrarenal RIs. In ischemic kidney (**a**) RIs (RI) are reduced if compared to the contralateral kidney (**b**), where vascular resistances are increased due to preglomerular barrage caused by systemic hypertension.

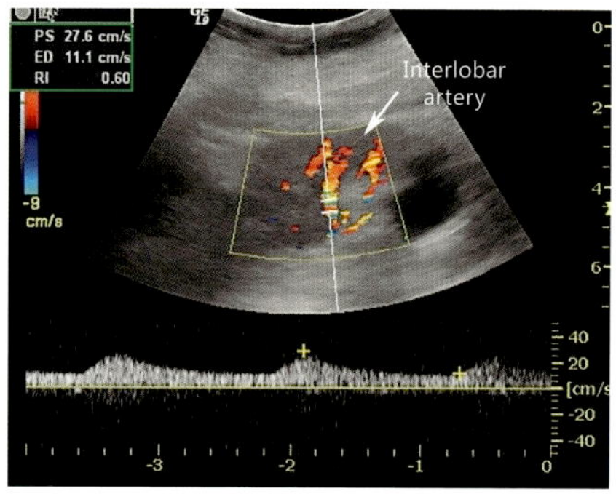

Fig. 4. Parvus-tardus sign. Spectral waveform shows a slow rise and a flattened systolic peak, downstream of a pre-occlusive stenosis. The parvus-tardus sign is an indirect sign of inflow resistance.

resistances increase due to the pre-glomerular barrage caused by systemic hypertension (fig. 3). In other words, RIs are low and lateralized in the ischemic kidney compared to the contralateral kidney. In case of severe stenosis (>80–85%), hilar arteries can show a slow and flattened curve (parvus-tardus sign) that indicates the lack of inflow and the fall of intrarenal resistances (fig. 4). In any case, RIs values in ischemic kidney vary according to age, impairment of microcirculation, parenchymal damage and therapy. In advanced kidney ischemia, when renal diameter is <9 cm and microcirculation remodeling prevails, RIs increase significantly (>0.75–0.80). Under such conditions, revascularization is contraindicated since there are poor chances of functional recovery [4].

Diseases of Medium Arteries and of Microcirculation

If ischemic nephropathy is due to a main damage of microcirculation, coronal kidney diameter is almost normal (10 to 10.5 cm) and parenchymal thickness is only slightly reduced, while there is a diffused and homogeneous hyperechoic

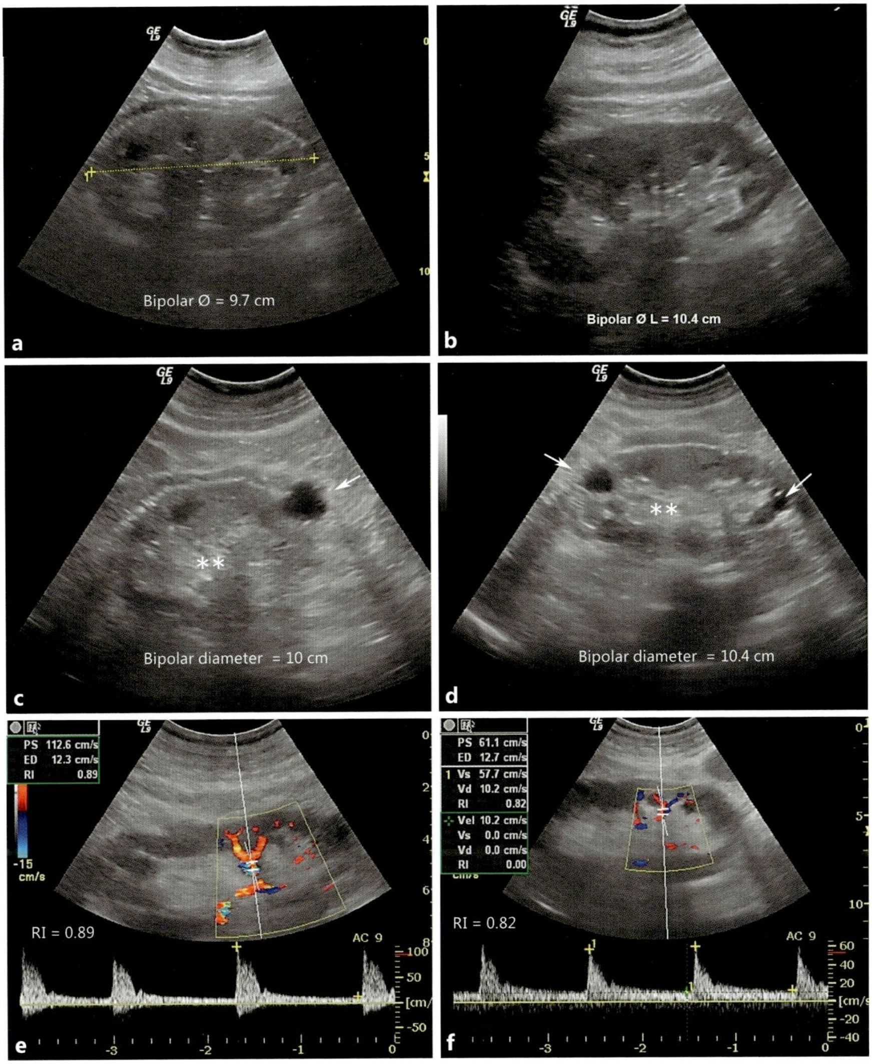

Fig. 5. Ischemic nephropathy caused by microcirculation damage. Kidney coronal diameter is almost normal (10–10.5 cm) (**a**, **b**), with reduced and hyperechoic parenchymal thickness, sinus sclerolipomatosis (**) and simple acquired cysts (**c**, **d**). **e**, **f** RIs show values >0.80 bilaterally, indicating a marked damage of microcirculation. ∅ = diameter. L = longitudinal.

aspect of renal cortex and medulla, often associated with sclerolipomatosis of the sinus and simple acquired cysts (fig. 5).

At CD, there are no significant changes in main renal artery velocity flow that could indicate a stenosis. Velocimetric complexes show an important gap between systolic and diastolic velocity with increased flow pulsatile component,

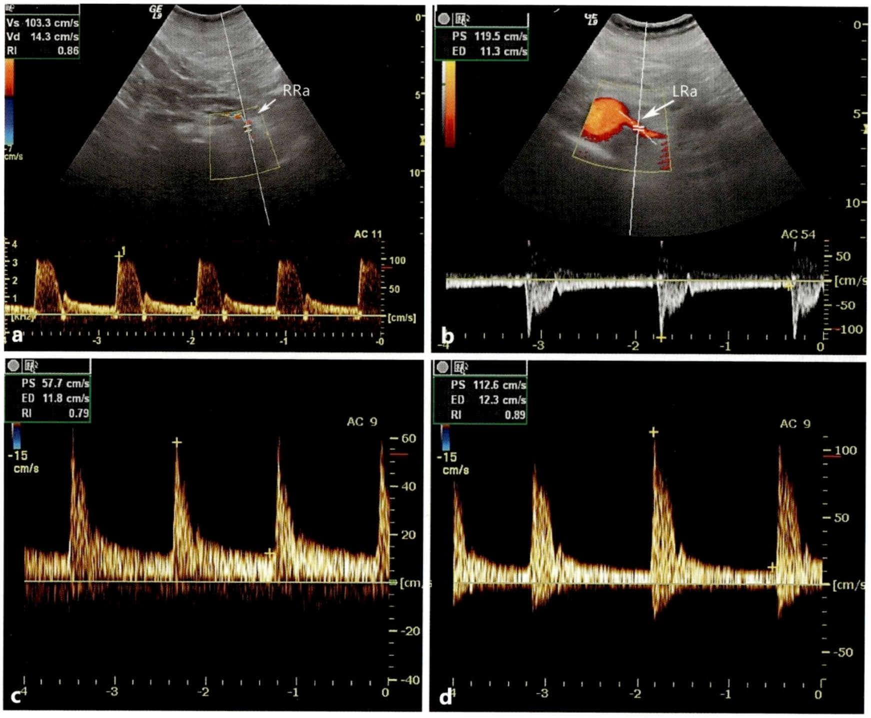

Fig. 6. Ischemic nephropathy with microcirculation involvement. Spectral curve in main renal artery (**a**, **b**) shows a marked gap between systolic and diastolic velocity (**c**, **d**). The increase of pulsatile flow, associated with a poor diastolic perfusion, is justified by the increase in stiffness and remodelling of small vessels. RRa = Renal right artery; LRa = left renal artery.

which means a reduced diastolic perfusion. This gap is due to a widespread increase in stiffness and vascular resistances (fig. 6) [5].

In some cases, kidney's morphology is almost normal and microcirculation involvement is revealed only by the increase of RIs values. Nephroangiosclerosis, as main artery stenosis, can be associated with atheroembolism, which can be spontaneous or induced by endovascular manoeuvres or anticoagulants. Migration of blood clots from atheromatous plaques in small parenchymal vessels causes acute kidney injury, which is often misdiagnosed. Atheroembolic disease contributes to chronic ischemic injury causing glomerular sclerohyalinosis and tubular atrophy.

From a morphological point of view, B-Mode US shows no specific sign of atheroembolic disease. In high-risk patients, it is common to find severe atheromasia (hyperechoic fibro-lipid plaques) of the abdominal aorta and large vessels (fig. 7). In classical atheroembolic disease, kidneys have a normal

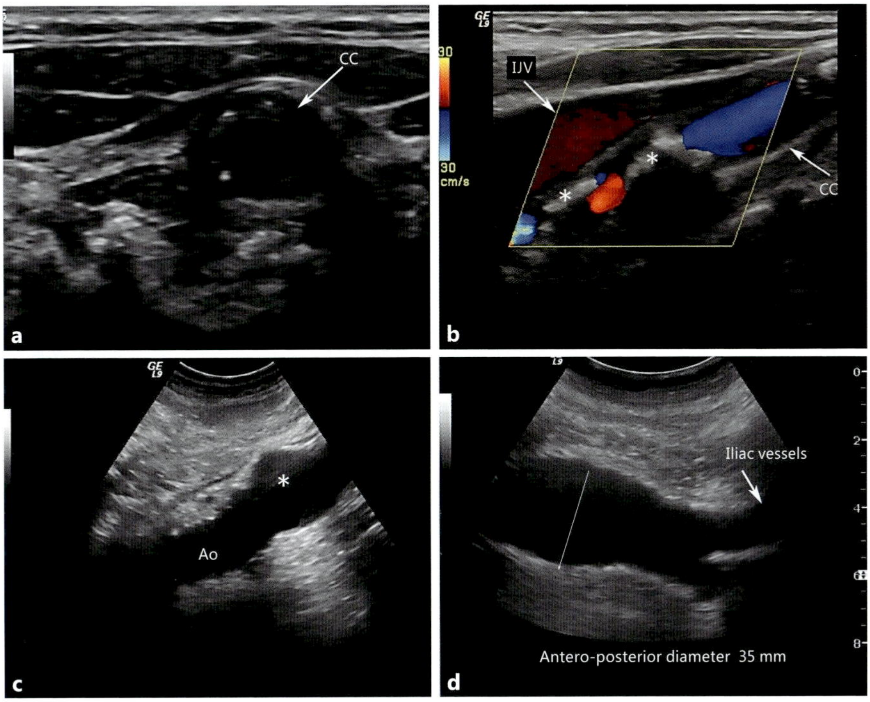

Fig. 7. Ischemic nephropathy with microcirculation involvement. B-Mode US does not show any specific sign of atheroembolic disease. In high-risk patients, a severe atheromasia of abdominal aorta or visceral vessels is common. **a** Transversal scan on the right common carotid artery shows an intima-media thickening and iso/hyperechoic atheromatous plaques. **b** Longitudinal scan on common carotid artery highlights the presence of flat and vegetating hyperechoic plaques along the vessel near wall (*). **c, d** Parasagittal median scan of the abdominal aorta: in both cases an atheromatous and aneurysmatic aorta is present. Ao = Aorta; * = anterior thrombosis; CC = common carotid artery; IJV = internal jugular vein.

structure, parenchyma may be hypoechoic or finely hyperechoic and renal profiles can be irregular due to the presence of scars. Clinical suspicion is suggested by patient case history and must be confirmed with laboratory and perfusion CD studies with or without contrast (contrast-enhanced US). As in nephroangiosclerosis, spectral curve shows a marked gap between systolic and diastolic velocity. Atheroembolism must be suspected in an elderly atherosclerotic patient with a rapid decrease of renal function, RIs >0.75–0.80 and eosinophilia after endovascular manoeuvres or anticoagulant therapy.

Conclusion

Vascular chronic diseases represent one of the leading causes of end-stage renal disease in incident dialysis patients. B-Mode US and CD have high sensitivity and specificity in the diagnosis of vascular chronic diseases. They should be, therefore, used to identify subjects in the high-risk population who are affected by stenosis of the main renal artery and to identify and characterize patients without RAS who have chronic ischemic nephropathy caused by nephroangiosclerosis and/or atheroembolic disease.

References

1 Lerman LO, Textor SC, Grande JP: Mechanisms of tissue injury in renal artery stenosis: ischemia and beyond. Prog Cardiovasc Dis 2009;52:196–203.

2 Wheatley K, Ives N, Gray R, Kalra PA, Moss JG, Baigent C, Carr S, Chalmers N, Eadington D, et al; ASTRAL Investigators: Revascularization versus medical therapy for renal-artery stenosis. N Engl J Med 2009;361: 1953–1962.

3 Cooper CJ, Murphy TP, Matsumoto A, Steffes M, Cohen DJ, Jaff M, Kuntz R, Jamerson K, Reid D, Rosenfield K, Rundback J, D'Agostino R, Henrich W, Dworkin L: Stent revascularization for the prevention of cardiovascular and renal events among patients with renal artery stenosis and systolic hypertension: rationale and design of the CORAL trial. Am Heart J 2006;152:59–66.

4 Radermacher J, Mengel M, Ellis S, et al: The renal arterial resistance index and renal allograft survival. N Engl J Med 2003;349:115–124.

5 Ikee R, Kobayashi S, Hemmi N, et al: Correlation between the resistive index by Doppler ultrasound and kidney function and histology. Am J Kidney Dis 2005;46:603–609.

Mario Meola, MD, PhD
Department of Internal Medicine
Sant'Anna School of Advanced Studies, University of Pisa
Via Savi 10, IT–56126 Pisa (Italy)
E-Mail mario.meola@unipi.it; m.meola@sssup.it

Meola M, Petrucci I, Ronco C (eds): Ultrasound Imaging in Acute and Chronic Kidney Disease.
Contrib Nephrol. Basel, Karger, 2016, vol 188, pp 89–97 (DOI: 10.1159/000445471)

Clinical Scenarios in Chronic Kidney Disease: Parenchymal Chronic Renal Diseases – Part 1

Ilaria Petrucci[a, b] · Sara Samoni[a, c] · Mario Meola[a, b]

[a]Sant'Anna School of Advanced Studies, Pisa, [b]Department of Internal Medicine, University of Pisa, Pisa, and [c]Department of Nephrology Dialysis and Transplantation, International Renal Research Institute (IRRIV), San Bortolo Hospital, Vicenza, Italy

Abstract

In diabetes, kidneys' morphological changes are non-specific at ultrasound (US) and they vary according to disease stage. In the earlier stages, kidneys are enlarged and diffusely hypoechoic due to hyperfiltration. Kidneys size decreases only in advanced stages whereas renal cortical echogenicity progressively increases due to glomerulosclerosis. Nephromegaly, as well as discrepancy between size and renal function, are typical features of diabetic nephropathy either in early or in advanced stages of the disease. Resistive indexes progressively increase together with serum creatinine levels and macro/microcirculation damage. Chronic glomerulonephritis (CGN) is the third leading cause of chronic kidney disease and it represents the clinical evolution of a variety of primary or secondary glomerular diseases. Kidneys in CGN are gradually reduced in volume, but remain symmetric, easily recognizable in renal space until the disease's later stages.

Kidney Damage in Diabetes Mellitus

Diabetes mellitus (DM) type 1 and 2 accelerates atherosclerotic damage of renal macro/microcirculation, and it is responsible for an evolving focal glomerulosclerosis. Intercurrent diseases such as urinary tract infections, acute papillary necrosis or renal artery stenosis can also enhance kidney damage caused by diabetes.

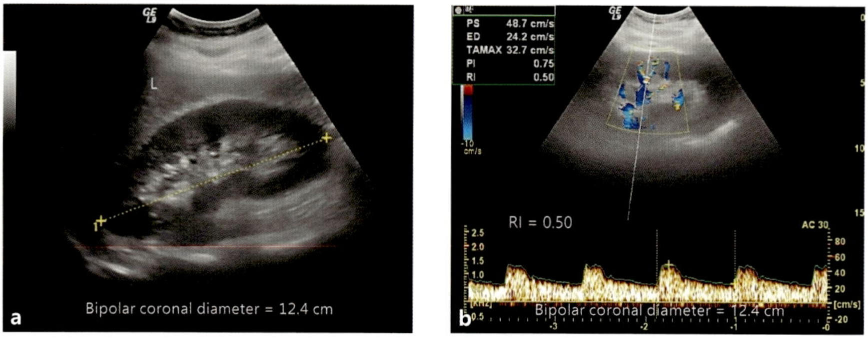

Fig. 1. Kidney and diabetes. Male, aged 54 years, with glucose intolerance, mild microalbuminuria and glycated hemoglobin 11.9%. **a** Nephromegaly due to poor metabolic control. **b** Renal hyperfiltration is demonstrated by low values of RIs (0.50–0.52).

At B-mode ultrasound (US), kidneys' structural aspect is non-specific and varies according to clinical conditions and disease stage. Kidney's increased volume and discrepancy between this morphological parameter and renal function are the hallmark of all disease stages and types [1, 2]. In pre-diabetes stage, kidneys are commonly increased in volume (longitudinal diameter >12–13 cm) and diffusely hypoechoic (fig. 1) [3]. Bilateral nephromegaly (bipolar coronal diameter >12 cm) is related to poor metabolic control and may be associated with abnormal values of glycated hemoglobin. Resistive indexes (RIs) in pre-diabetes stage are often symmetrically reduced (<0.60), as they reflect kidney's hyperfiltration (fig. 1).

Diffused hypoechogenicity highlights parenchymal structure, and kidneys are easily recognizable if compared to other retroperitoneal surrounding structures. Kidney profiles, urinary tract characteristics and morphology of the renal papillae may be altered by intercurrent episodes of pyelonephritis or acute papillary necrosis. During the acute phase (colic pain and infection), US reveals no specific signs of papillary necrosis. In later stages, US excludes the presence of stones and can highlight hydronephrosis with ureteral obstruction. In one-third of cases, detached necrotic papilla remains in the pelvis, near the medulla and the dilated calyces [4] (fig. 2).

Nephromegaly is a morphological feature that characterizes diabetic nephropathy in all clinical conditions, even if morpho-functional discrepancy is less perceived in early stages than in advanced stages (fig. 3). In type-1 diabetes, the increase in volume correlates with the degree of albuminuria and this correlation becomes more significant as proteinuria increases [5].

The correlation between volume increase and albuminuria is also evident in type 2 diabetes [6]. In overt diabetic nephropathy, RIs increase when kidneys begin to decrease in volume and microalbuminuria appears [7]. In a study on a

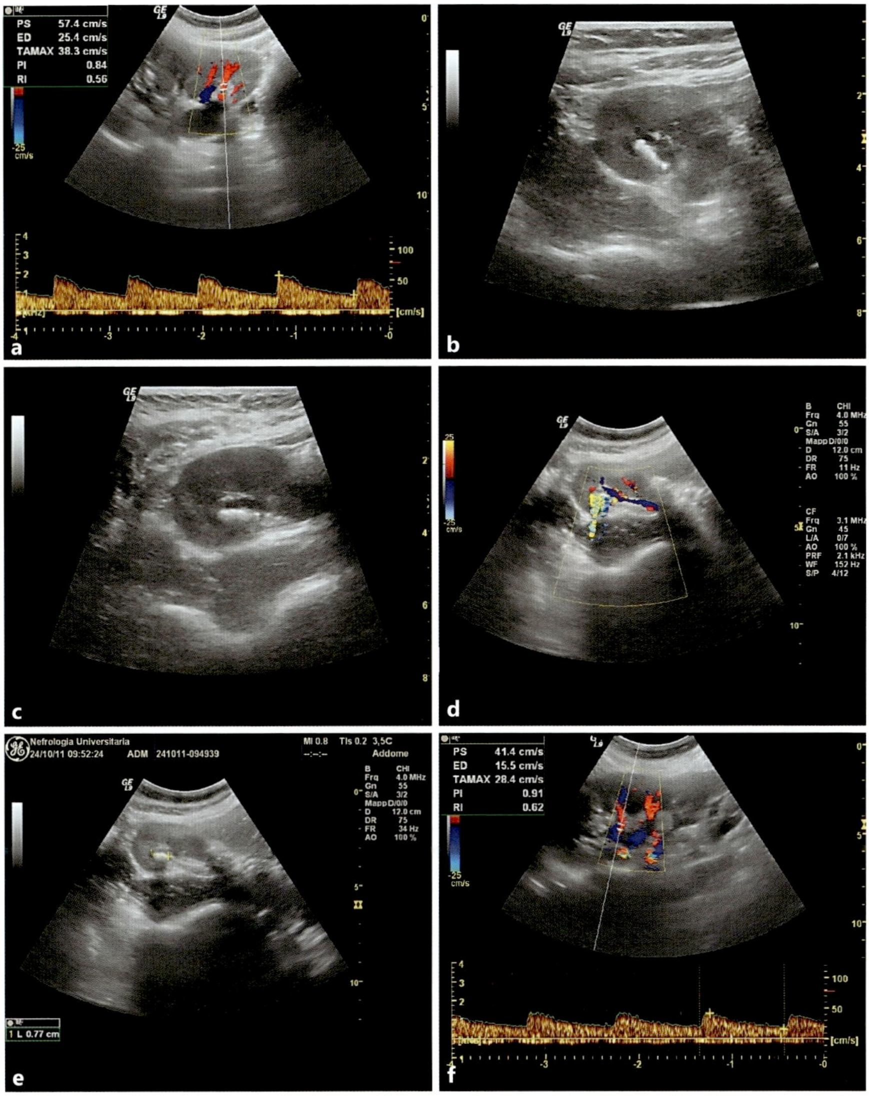

Fig. 2. Kidney and diabetes. Female, aged 25 years, type 1 diabetes since the age of 10 years, with right kidney multiple lithiasis associated with recurrent infections and treated with lithotomy. Normal renal function, no microalbuminuria. **a** Right kidney with pelvis' hypotonia and RIs of 0.56. **b**, **c** Evidence of a superior polar cavitation with amorphous calcified material (amputated papilla secondary to papillary necrosis, confirmed at urography). **d**, **e** Inferior calyceal lithiasis. **f** Left nephromegaly with prominent lobulations with RIs of 0.62.

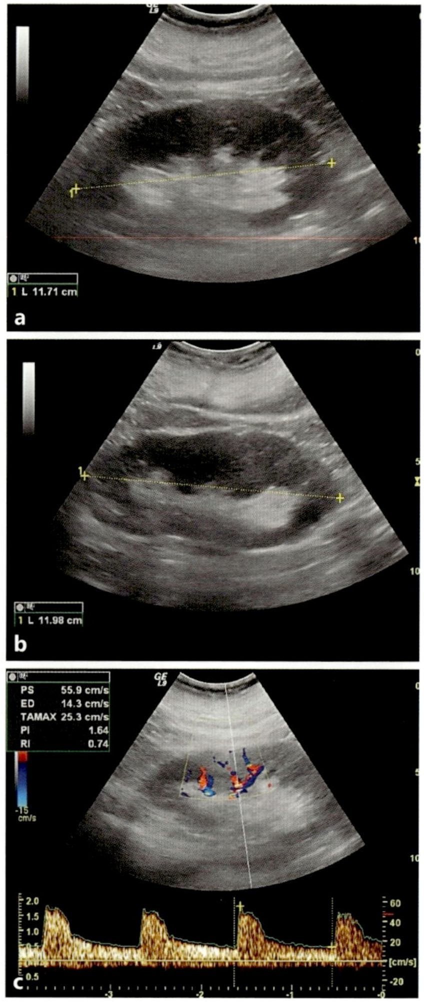

Fig. 3. Kidney and diabetes. Overt diabetic nephropathy. Female, aged 68 years, with 19 years of type 2 diabetes. Serum creatinine 4.3 mg/dl, creatinine clearance 19 ml/min, proteinuria 2.4 g/day. (**a**, **b**) Nephromegaly and (**c**) V/t curve with an important gap between systolic and diastolic velocity due to increased microcirculation resistance. RIs are 0.74.

large series of patients with overt diabetic nephropathy, Ishimura et al. [8] evaluated the correlation between RIs values and intima-media thickness of the common carotid artery and of the superficial femoral artery, demonstrating a clear correlation between these parameters and the progression of vascular damage.

Moreover, study population, stratified according to the value of serum creatinine (sCr), showed a progressive growth of RIs related to the disease's stage. In patients with sCr >3.4 mg/dl (chronic kidney disease [CKD] stage 4) RIs were 0.85 ± 0.05, while in control patients RIs were 0.66 ± 0.04. In patients with decreased renal function (CKD 2,3) RIs values ranged from 0.69 ± 0.05 to 0.74 ± 0.06 (fig. 4) [8]. When chronic structural alterations are evident, RIs still increase

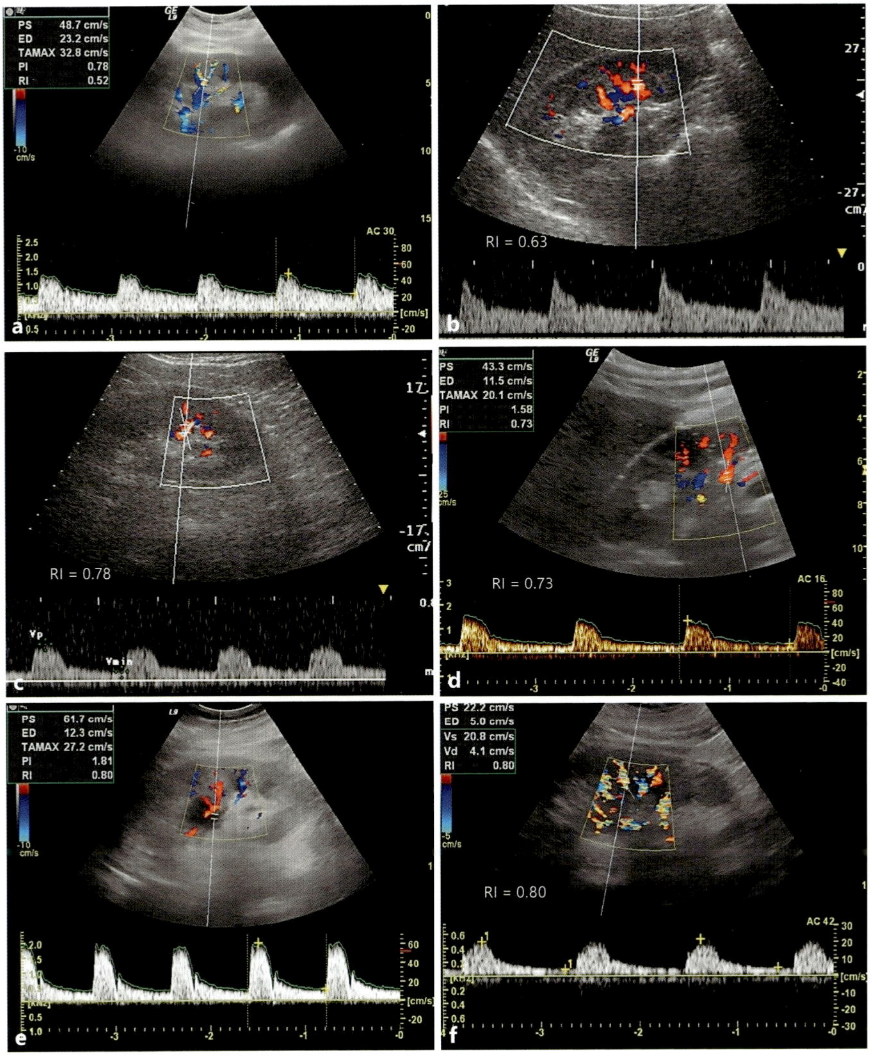

Fig. 4. Diabetic nephropathy and intraparenchymal RIs. Intraparenchymal RI progression in right kidney (**a**, **c**, **e**) and left kidney (**b**, **d**, **f**) is related to the functional stage of diabetic nephropathy. Increased stiffness and microcirculation remodelling are pathological aspects that affect systemic and renal circulation. Vascular bed reduction justifies the progressive increase in pulsatile flow and, consequently, continuous diastolic flow is dispersed in the Winkessel system.

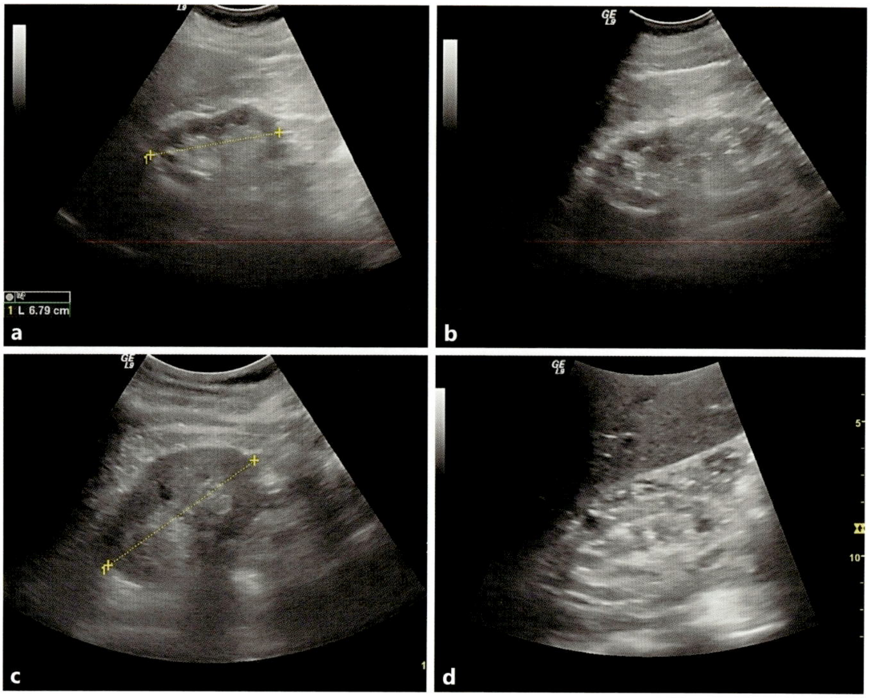

Fig. 5. End-stage kidney caused by primary CGN. Kidneys' morphology in end-stage CGN is preserved until the later stages of CKD, despite the progressive volume reduction. End-stage kidneys due to mesangial proliferative glomerulonephritis (**a**), post-infectious glomerulonephritis (**b**), IgA nephropathy (**c**) and focal sclerosis (**d**).

showing a clear correlation with the decrease in glomerular filtration rate (GFR) and severity of systemic vascular damage. In this stage, main renal artery flow bilaterally acquires a pulsatile pattern, due to the irreversible increase in parenchymal vascular impedance.

Kidney Damage in Chronic Glomerulonephritis

Chronic glomerulonephritis (CGN) is the third leading cause of CKD and it represents the clinical evolution of many primary and secondary glomerular diseases. Kidneys in CGN are gradually reduced in volume, but remain symmetric, easily recognizable in renal space until the disease's later stages (fig. 5). End-stage kidneys' profiles are often unrecognizable and the structural aspect of parenchyma becomes indefinite and amorphous. This happens especially in the left side where, due to the lack of the acoustic liver window, kidney often becomes indistinguishable from peri/pararenal fat. Typically, normal respira-

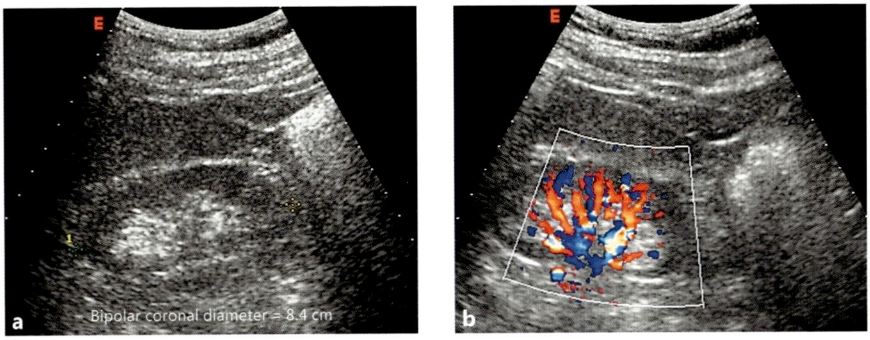

Fig. 6. End-stage kidney caused by membranoproliferative glomerulonephritis. Pre-dialysis CKD stage 5. (**a**) Kidney shows a marked volume reduction, but profiles are relatively irregular. Parenchymal blushing at color Doppler (**b**) is still present and less compromised if compared with end-stage kidneys with vascular or tubulointerstitial damage.

tory kidney movements, the presence of multiple small cysts and/or parenchymal nephrocalcinosis help to identify end-stage kidney. Rarely, hypoechoic perirenal fat surrounding the end-stage kidney can simulate a perirenal collection. In CKD with nephrotic syndrome resistant to medical treatments, kidneys' structure looks more like acute forms: kidneys are increased in volume, globular, with hypoechoic and edematous pyramids until the disease reaching the later stages or proteinuria is not spontaneously reduced.

Color Doppler (CD) sampling shows a parallel behaviour, which means that it highlights a progressive impairment of parenchymal blushing as blood flow and GFR lower, although the reduction in perfusion is less severe than in other forms of parenchymal disease (fig. 6). In end stages, renal perfusion disappears or is not evident even with low pulse repetition frequency values. Main artery and interlobar vessels spectral waveform preserve low-resistance morphology until the end stages, even if it shows a progressive fall in amplitude and diastolic flow. RIs increase very slowly and they reach or exceed values of 0.70 only in end stages (fig. 7) [9]. This parameter, although non-specific, distinguishes CGN from vasculitis, nephrosclerosis and end-stage chronic interstitial nephropathy with or without reflux. From a pathophysiological point of view, the trend of RIs in CGN is justified by several conditions: (1) glomeruli that receive the great part of renal blood flow represent <10% of the total renal volume, (2) gradual amputation of sclerotic glomeruli causes a short circuit of blood from the afferent vessel to the efferent artery and (3) primary glomerular diseases prevail in young and adults, or in people who have not yet undergone a dystrophic wall remodelling of microcirculation. In fact, in patients with CGN, RIs tend to decrease after administration of inhibitors of angiotensin 1 and 2 receptors and calcium chan-

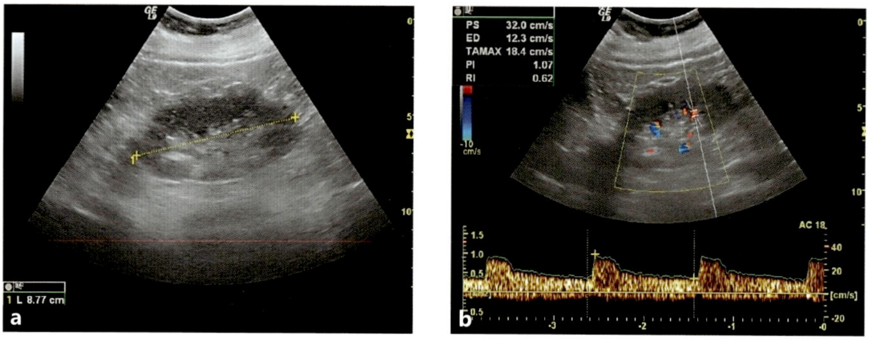

Fig. 7. CGN and renal perfusion. Pre-dialysis CKD stage 5 secondary to proliferative CGN. Hypertension treated with ACE inhibitors. In CGN, RIs increase slowly and reach values of 0.62 only in advanced stages (**a**, **b**).

nel blockers. This happens even in diabetic nephropathy and in acute hypertensive nephrosclerosis, and it justifies the renoprotective action of renin-angiotensin system inhibitors [10, 11]. These findings provide evidence that in CGN caused by glomerular damage, vasomotility and capacitance of renal microcirculation are preserved despite the progression of glomerular injury. RIs reach higher values only in advanced disease stages, when glomerulosclerosis is associated with a diffused interstitial and vascular fibrosis.

Conclusion

In diabetes, US and CD are useful in disease staging and clinical follow-up. US and CD features vary depending on disease stage. Nephromegaly and discrepancy between this morphological parameter and renal function are the hallmark of all disease stages and types. RIs reflect kidney's hyperfiltration in the early stages and then they increase in overt diabetic nephropathy. When chronic structural alterations are evident, RIs increase showing a clear correlation with the decrease in GFR and severity of systemic vascular damage. On the other hand, US and CD are useful in characterizing CGN because kidneys are gradually reduced in volume, but remain symmetric, easily recognizable in renal space until the disease's later stages. CD sampling highlights a progressive parenchymal blushing impairment as blood flow and GFR lower, although the reduction in perfusion is less severe than in any other form of parenchymal disease.

References

1 Segel MC, Lecky JW, Slasky BS: Diabetes mellitus: the predominant cause of bilateral renal enlargement. Radiology 1984;153:341–342.

2 Banholzer P, Haslbeck M, Edelmann E, Sager P, Staudigl K, Mehnert H: [Sonographic changes in the size of the kidneys in type I diabetes as a method of early detection of diabetic nephropathy]. Ultraschall Med 1988;9: 255–259.

3 Christiansen JS, Gammelgaard J, Frandsen M, Parving HH: Increased kidney size, glomerular filtration rate and renal plasma flow in short-term insulin-dependent diabetics. Diabetologia 1981;20:451–456.

4 Vijayaraghavan SB, Kandasamy SV, Mylsamy A, Prabhakar M: Sonographic features of necrosed renal papillae causing hydronephrosis. J Ultrasound Med 2003;22:951–956; quiz 957–958.

5 Feldt-Rasmussen B, Hegedüs L, Mathiesen ER, Deckert T: Kidney volume in type 1 (insulin-dependent) diabetic patients with normal or increased urinary albumin excretion: effect of long-term improved metabolic control. Scand J Clin Lab Invest 1991;51:31–36.

6 Derchi LE, Martinoli C, Saffioti S, Pontremoli R, De Micheli A, Bordone C: Ultrasonographic imaging and Doppler analysis of renal changes in non-insulin-dependent diabetes mellitus. Acad Radiol 1994;1:100–105.

7 Marzano MA, Pompili M, Rapaccini GL, et al: Early renal involvement in diabetes mellitus: comparison of renal Doppler US and radioisotope evaluation of glomerular hyperfiltration. Radiology 1998;209:813–817.

8 Ishimura E, Nishizawa Y, Kawagishi T, Okuno Y, Kogawa K, Fukumoto S, Maekawa K, Hosoi M, Inaba M, Emoto M, Morii H: Intrarenal hemodynamic abnormalities in diabetic nephropathy measured by duplex Doppler sonography. Kidney Int 1997;51:1920–1927.

9 Platt JF, Rubin JM, Ellis JH, et al: Duplex Doppler US of the kidney: differentiation of obstructive from nonobstructive dilatation. Radiology 1989;171:515–517.

10 Watanabe S, Okura T, Kurata M, et al: Valsartan reduces serum cystatin C and the renal vascular resistance in patients with essential hypertension. Clin Exp Hypertens 2006;28: 451–461.

11 Leoncini G, Martinoli C, Viazzi F, et al: Changes in renal resistive index and urinary albumin excretion in hypertensive patients under long-term treatment with lisinopril or nifedipine GITS. Nephron 2002;90:169–173.

Mario Meola, MD, PhD
Department of Internal Medicine
Sant'Anna School of Advanced Studies, University of Pisa
Via Savi 10, IT–56126 Pisa (Italy)
E-Mail mario.meola@unipi.it; m.meola@sssup.it

Meola M, Petrucci I, Ronco C (eds): Ultrasound Imaging in Acute and Chronic Kidney Disease.
Contrib Nephrol. Basel, Karger, 2016, vol 188, pp 98–107 (DOI: 10.1159/000445472)

Clinical Scenarios in Chronic Kidney Disease: Parenchymal Chronic Renal Diseases – Part 2

Ilaria Petrucci[a, b] · Sara Samoni[a, c] · Mario Meola[a, b]

[a]Sant'Anna School of Advanced Studies, Pisa, [b]Department of Internal Medicine, University of Pisa, Pisa, and [c]Department of Nephrology Dialysis and Transplantation, International Renal Research Institute (IRRIV), San Bortolo Hospital, Vicenza, Italy

Abstract

Secondary nephropathies can be associated with disreactive immunological disorders or with a non-inflammatory glomerular damage. In systemic lupus erythematosus (SLE), scleroderma and rheumatoid arthritis as in other connective tissue diseases, kidney volume and cortex echogenicity are the parameters that best correlate with clinical severity of the disease, even if the morphological aspect is generally non-specific. Doppler studies in SLE document the correlation between resistance indexes (RIs) values and renal function. Acquired immunodeficiency syndrome (HIV) causes different types of renal damage. At ultrasound (US), kidneys have almost a normal volume, while during superinfection they enlarge (coronal diameter >13 cm) and become globular, loosing their normal aspect. Cortex appears highly hyperechoic, uniform or patchy. Microcalcifications of renal cortex and medulla are a US sign that can suggest HIV. In amyloidosis, kidneys appear normal or increased in volume in the early stages of disease. Renal cortex is diffusely hyperechoic and pyramids can show normal size and morphology, but more often they appear poorly defined and hyperechoic. RIs are very high since the early stages of the disease. Nephromegaly with normal kidney shape is the first sign of lymphoma or multiple myeloma. In systemic vasculitis, renal cortex is diffusely hyperechoic, while pyramids appear hypoechoic and globular due to interstitial edema. When vasculitis determines advanced chronic kidney disease stages, kidneys show no specific signs. Microcirculation damage is highlighted by increased RIs values >0.70 in the chronic phase.

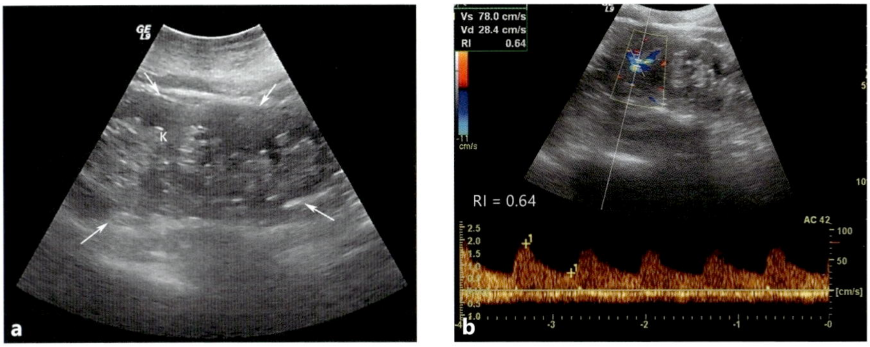

Fig. 1. Chronic interstitial nephropathy associated with Sjogren's syndrome. Female, aged 82 years with a 30-year history of Sjogren's disease. Serum creatinine 2.2 mg/dl, CKD stage 4. End-stage right kidney. Left kidney: longitudinal diameter 11 cm, duplicated collecting and arterial system. **a** Parenchyma is diffusely hyperechoic and corticomedullar differentiation is lost. Presence of multiple hyperechoic medullary and cortical spots. **b** Intraparenchymal RIs of 0.64. No evidence of renal artery stenosis. K = Kidney.

Secondary Nephropathies

Secondary nephropathies can be associated with disreactive immunological disorders (systemic lupus erythematosus [SLE], bacterial endocarditis, chronic B or C hepatitis, acquired immunodeficiency syndrome [HIV] infection) or with a non-inflammatory glomerular damage (amyloidosis, Hodgkin's disease, HIV infection, heroin toxicity, drug toxicity, neoplasms).

Immunological Secondary Glomerulonephritis

In SLE, scleroderma and rheumatoid arthritis as in other connective tissue diseases, kidney volume and cortex echogenicity are the parameters that best correlate with clinical severity of the disease, even if the morphological aspect is generally non-specific and does not allow characterizing the histological damage (fig. 1) [1]. Doppler studies in SLE document the correlation between resistance indexes (RIs) values and renal function but they are not useful to characterize the stages of lupus nephritis (fig. 2) [2].

HIV causes different types of renal damage [3]. The most severe forms of proteinuria or nephrotic syndrome occur in blacks and the histological damage is a focal collapsing glomerulosclerosis HIV related or, more rarely, a membranous/membranous proliferative glomerulonephritis or a minimal change disease. Immunodeficiency and CD4 deficit may cause chronic kidney damage by favouring opportunistic infections (histoplasmosis, Pneumocystis carinii,

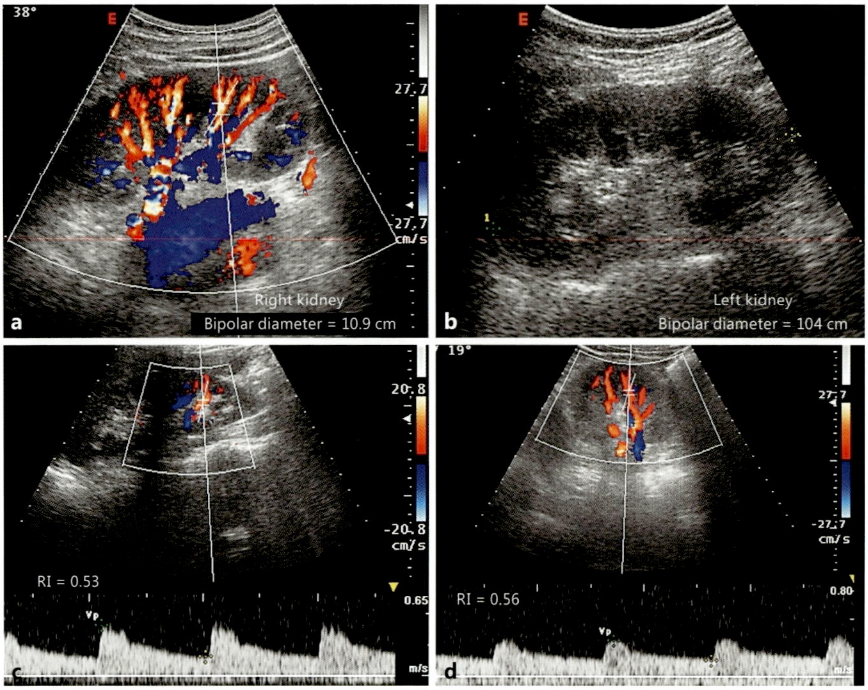

Fig. 2. Lupus nephritis stage 2. Mesangial glomerulonephritis type 2b. Mesangial damage due to deposition of immunoglobulins prevails in this stage, associated with microangiopathy with ischemic and thrombotic sclerosis. Kidney appears well perfused (**a**). Renal volume is normal, corticomedullar profiles are poorly defined and there is a widespread hypoechogenicity (**b**). The absence of vasculitis is demonstrated by low RIs values in both kidneys (**c**, **d**).

intracellular Mycobacterium avium, fungal infections, etc.). Chronic damage can be induced by a chronic interstitial nephritis induced by highly active antiretroviral drugs (tenofovir, indinavir) or by antibacterial drugs used for the treatment of opportunistic infections (amphotericin, cotrimoxazole). A lymphoma or a Kaposi's sarcoma can injure kidneys, although the latter is located mostly in the lower urinary tract. Finally, antiretroviral drugs can cause a vascular damage (renal artery stenosis, hemolytic uremic syndrome, acute renal failure), which determines a chronic renal damage.

At ultrasound (US), kidneys have almost a normal volume, while in 20% of cases (often during superinfection) they enlarge (coronal diameter >13 cm) and become globular, loosing their normal aspect [4, 5]. In 89% of cases, cortex appears highly hyperechoic, uniform or patchy, similar to that of the renal sinus and more hyperechoic than the liver [6]. Some authors suggest that uniform or patchy hyperechogenicity and the loss of the parenchymal differentiation associated with an increase in volume are strongly suggestive of HIV-related nephropathy, even if there is no correlation between the degree of hyperechogenicity and renal damage [7]. Sometimes, cortical damage is associated with a pielo-ureteral wall thickening. Nevertheless, this sign is sometimes evident even in upper urinary tract infections and in acute tubular necrosis but, in any case, pielo-ureteral wall thickening and cortical widespread hyperechogenicity should suggest the possibility of an HIV nephropathy [8]. 50% of patients with HIV show an apparent reduction of renal sinus fat due to the presence of edema more than to the real reduction in adipose tissue [9]. Dense and diffuse microcalcifications of renal cortex and medulla are a US sign that can suggest HIV. This structural finding is common in HIV patients with a superimposed infection with Mycobacterium avium, Pneumocystis carinii or histoplasmosis [4]. In patients with active disease, renal bacterial and fungal infections may occur. Patients with HIV also have a very high risk of renal lymphoma [4].

Non-Inflammatory Glomerular Damage

Amyloidosis is a thesaurismosis characterized by the deposition of insoluble fibrillar proteinaceous material in the extracellular matrix. The name *amyloid* comes from a mistaken identification of the substance as starch based on crude iodine-staining techniques. Fibrils have a variable chemical composition; they are identified by apple-green birefringence when stained with congo red and seen under polarized light. The outermost part of amyloid (95% of the substance) comes from a specific protein, while a globular glycoprotein of the basement membranes (P amyloid) forms the core. Disease may be systemic or localized, and it is classified according to the amyloid chemical structure [10]. Macroscopically, amyloid appears albumoid, smooth and translucent, like hyaline substance. Spleen, kidney, heart, brain, liver and gastrointestinal tract are the organs that can be affected by amyloidosis. From a clinical point of view, amyloidosis can be primary or idiopathic (not associated with other medical conditions), familiar and, finally, secondary to chronic inflammatory diseases or cancer. Systemic idiopathic amyloidosis or amyloidosis associated with multiple myeloma are the most common forms of amyloidosis and they are characterized by the deposition of light chains k and λ (AL amyloid), followed by secondary inflammatory/reactive amyloidosis characterized by deposition of amyloid AA. This form of amyloidosis is associated with aging, chronic infectious diseases (tuberculosis, bronchiectasis, osteomyelitis, leprosy), inflammatory diseases (rheumatoid arthritis, granulomatous ileitis), Hodgkin's disease, other cancers and familial Mediterranean fever. The third type of amyloidosis (familiar forms

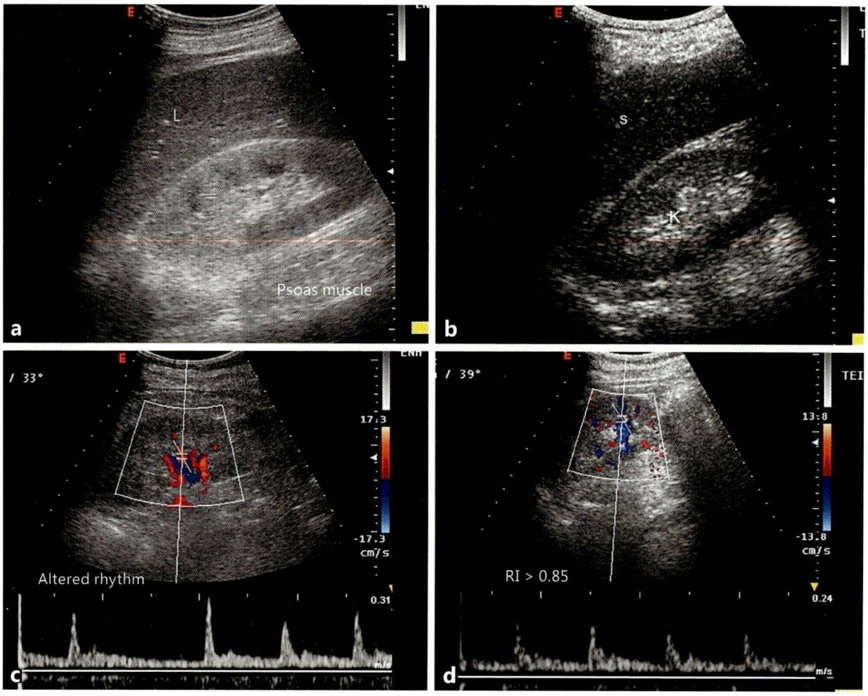

Fig. 3. Kidney amyloidosis. Male, aged 54 years, with light chain myeloma (λ chains), nephrotic proteinuria (2.6 g/day) and preserved renal function (serum creatinine 1–1.2 mg/dl). Histological diagnosis: amyloidosis. Periumbilical fat biopsy showed a positive result with alkaline Congo red staining. **a, b** Kidneys have a normal volume, but they appear hyperechoic. Corticomedullary feature is altered and medulla is diffusely hyperechoic. **c, d** Unlike in nephrotic syndrome due to minimal changes disease, membranous or membrane proliferative glomerulonephritis, pyramids are not hypoechoic. Parenchymal perfusion is preserved but RIs are very high (0.85). K = Kidney; L = liver, S = spleen.

not associated with other diseases) is characterized by neuropathy, nephropathy and cardiac disease. Altogether, these forms represent about 85% of cases of amyloidosis. All of them are characterized by glomerular deposition of amyloid substance that causes a progressive renal sclerosis.

At US, kidneys appear normal or increased in volume in the early stages of disease, when renal function is preserved and only proteinuria is present. Renal cortex is diffusely hyperechoic due to amyloid deposits and pyramids can show normal size and morphology, but more often they appear poorly defined and hyperechoic (fig. 3). Sometimes, heterogeneous, hypoechoic and edematous pyramids can accompany hyperechoic cortex. This is less common and occurs in systemic amyloidosis associated with nephrotic syndrome (approximately 5% of patients with rheumatoid arthritis) [11]. According to disease duration and severity, kidneys may be reduced in volume and they become small and sclerotic. Structural kidney features in advanced stages become indistinguishable from other forms of CKD, when glomerular and interstitial sclerosis with tubular atrophy prevails. RIs are very high since the early stages of the disease (>0.75–0.80) (fig. 3).

Lymphoma involves the kidney in 2–6% of cases because of a diffuse lymphocytic infiltration of the interstitium, a secondary glomerulopathy, a urinary tract obstruction or a toxic action of chemotherapy. Minimal change disease is the most common glomerulopathy (fig. 4), while focal and segmental glomerulosclerosis, membranous glomerulonephritis and mesangial proliferative nephropathy are observed more rarely. All forms of renal involvement may lead to end-stage CKD. Primitive renal lymphoma is very rare (1% of cases), because kidneys' lymphomatous infiltration is usually an extranodal location of systemic non-Hodgkin's lymphoma [12]. Renal involvement may be unilateral or bilateral, focal, multifocal, diffuse or associated with a perirenal lymphomatous mass. In nephrology, the most interesting form is the less common one, that is, the Burkitt's lymphoma and acute lymphoblastic leukemia infiltrative form. Nephromegaly with normal kidney shape is the first sign of renal lymphocytic interstitial infiltration. At US, the presence of irregular and diffused hypoechoic parenchymal areas and, sometimes, the loss of normal sinus echogenicity may suggest the diagnosis of lymphoma. In some cases, kidney's infiltration is so widespread that it destroys the parenchyma, so kidney at US appears as a large amorphous, hypoechoic and poorly perfused mass [13].

Patients refer to clinicians because of acute kidney injury resulting from the destruction of the normal renal architecture, especially if the disease affects both kidneys. In these cases, contrast-enhanced CT, despite the fall in GFR, is pivotal to asses disease staging and to document structural kidney alterations (inhomogeneous enhancement, loss of normal structural pattern between cortex and medulla, infiltration of renal sinus, compression and dislocation of the excretory system) [14]. In any case, the presence of atypical lymphocytes at cytology or histology confirms the diagnosis, because in normal kidneys lymphocytes are not present. Differential diagnosis of infiltrating and diffused lymphomas must consider other diseases such as invasive transitional cell carcinoma of the pelvis or medullar ducts and severe pyelonephritis if fever is present.

In multiple myeloma, as in other lymphoproliferative disorders, renal involvement may appear with proteinuria, nephrotic syndrome and/or acute or chronic renal failure. Kidney damage in myeloma is due to the abnormal proliferation of plasma cells and to the presence of circulating paraproteins and/or light chains. Light chains easily pass through the glomerular filter so they are reabsorbed and metabolized in the proximal tubule. The exceeding light chains saturate the reabsorption mechanism; they damage renal tubules, favour cylinders' formation and can be deposited in the glomerulus. Therefore, renal

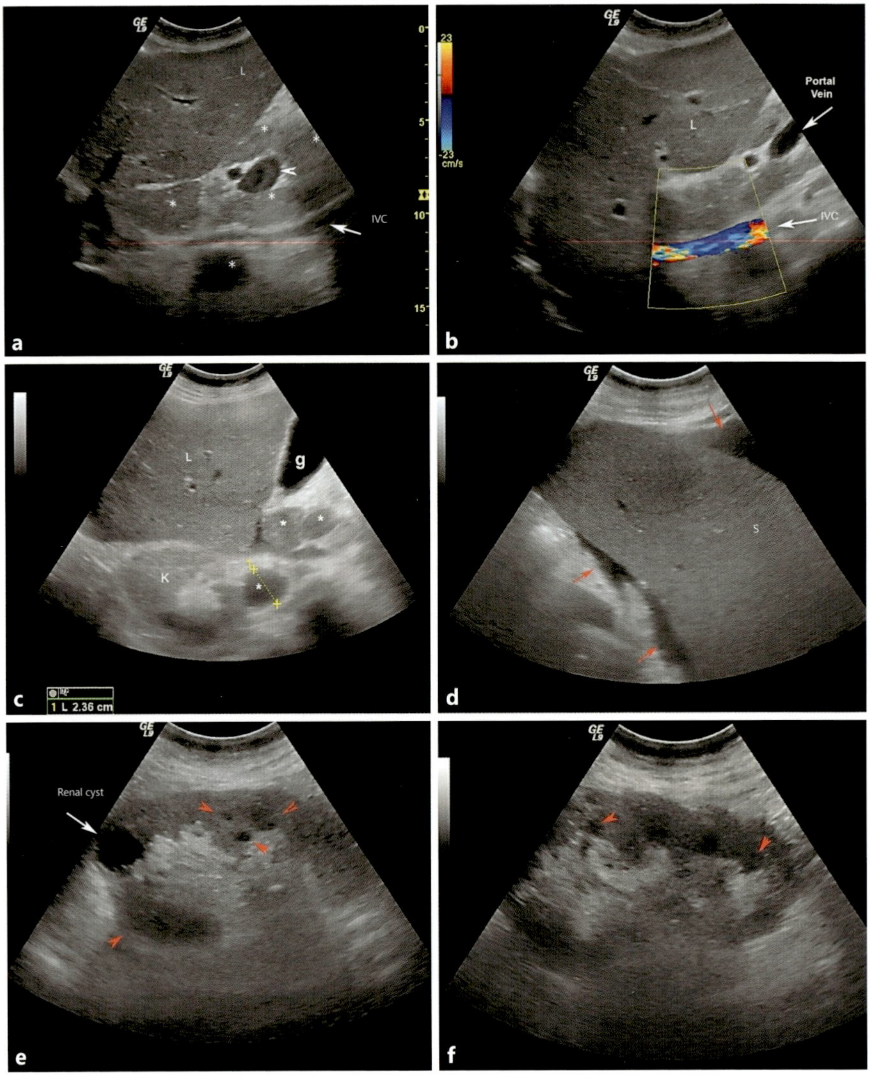

Fig. 4. Minimal change glomerulonephritis associated with systemic non-Hodgkin lymphoma. Male, aged 73 years with anemia, asthenia, nephrotic syndrome and retroperitoneal and perirenal right lymphoadenopathy. Serum creatinine 1.0 mg/dl, proteinuria 17 g/day, anasarcatic state. **a**, **b** Longitudinal paramedian right scan that shows a hyperecoic liver with right lobe diameter of 14.8 cm and coarse and multiple confluent lymphoadenopathy in the hilar region, paracaval and perirenal space (**c**). **d** Splenomegaly (longitudinal diameter >18 cm) with perisplenic effusion (red arrow). **e**, **f** Kidneys are increased in volume, with hyperechoic pyramids. Small and diffused hypoechoic lesions are present into the renal parenchyma (red arrowhead) and they are related to cellular infiltration. Arrow = Renal cyst; L = liver; S = spleen; K = right kidney; g = gallbladder; * = lymphoadenopathy; IVC = inferior vena cava.

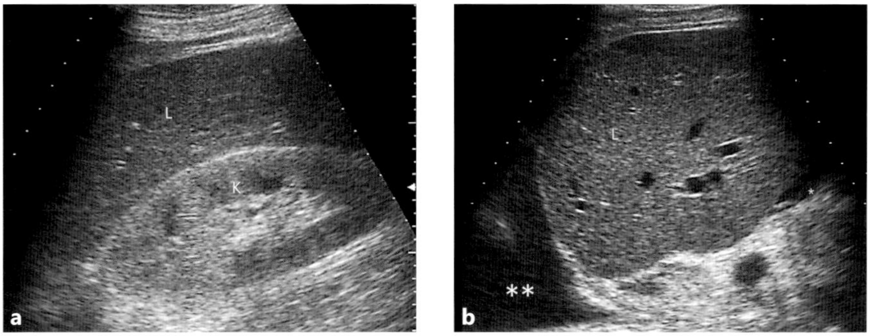

Fig. 5. Kidney and mixed cryoglobulinemia. Cryoglobulinemic nephropathy is a vasculitis commonly related to Hepatitis C virus infection. Histological renal feature reflects a membrane-proliferative glomerulonephritis. **a** Kidneys are increased in volume, hyperechoic, with more or less irregular pyramids. Kidneys' aspect is associated with chronic hepatopathy, portal hypertension and splenomegaly. If nephrotic syndrome is present, pleural and abdominal effusion can be evidenced (**b**). * = Effusion in the Morrison's space; ** = pleural effusion; L = liver; K = kidney.

involvement in myeloma (myeloma kidney) may be due to tubular obstruction and tubular lesions caused by light chains (cast nephropathy), to paraprotein glomerular deposition (AL amyloidosis disease and light chain nephropathy) or, finally, to chronic interstitial damage caused by hypercalcemia, hyperuricemia, dehydration, drug toxicity and iodinated contrast [15]. At US, kidney volume and cortical echogenicity are the parameters that best correlate with clinical severity, as in other chronic diseases, but morphological features are generally non-specific and do not define the type of damage; so renal biopsy is needed [16].

Renal involvement during systemic vasculitis is very common. The term 'vasculitis' includes polyarteritis nodosa, Wegener's granulomatosis with polyangiitis, micropolyarteritis, Churg-Strauss syndrome, Burger's disease, Behcet's syndrome, arteritis of Takayasu and hypersensitivity vasculitis (Henoch-Schonlein purpura, mixed cryoglobulinemia) [17]. The most common clinical renal manifestations of vasculitis are acute renal failure and blood hypertension due to renal ischemia induced by activation of the renin-angiotensin system. In any case, morphological renal features are non-specific at US, either in acute or in chronic damage, so renal biopsy is mandatory. In acute phase, the most important US sign is the morpho-functional discrepancy, that is, renal coronal diameters and parenchymal thickness (16–18 mm) are normal while renal function is impaired (fig. 5).

Renal cortex is diffusely hyperechoic, while pyramids appear hypoechoic and globular due to interstitial edema, as in other acute kidney diseases. In some situations, diffuse hyperechoic parenchyma with loss of parenchymal differentiation can prevail. In some rare cases, renal morphology can be completely normal.

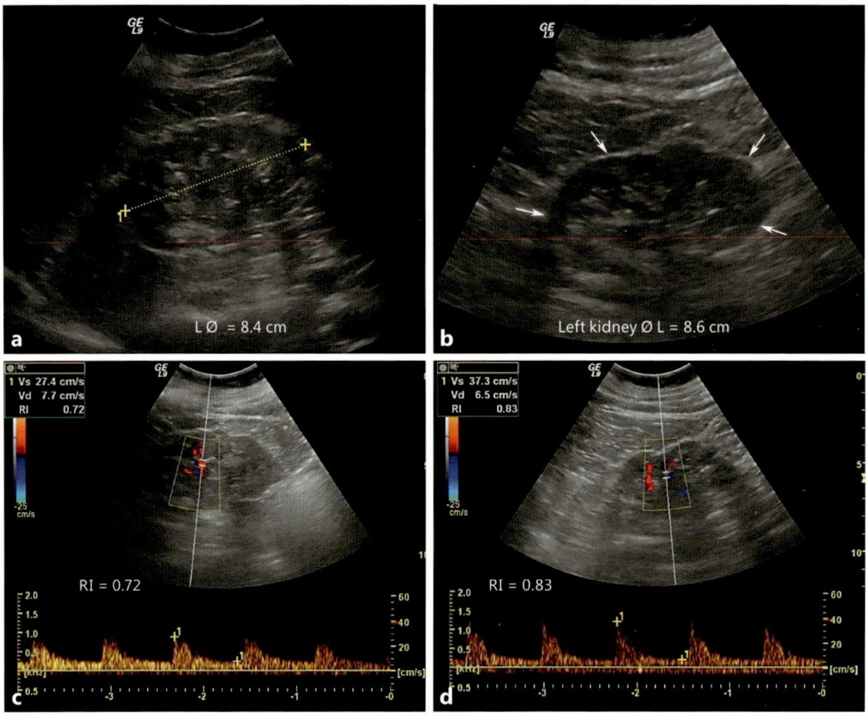

Fig. 6. Kidney and mixed cryoglobulinemia. Progression to end stage CKD is uncommon. Female, aged 67 years, with a membranoproliferative glomerulonephritis diagnosed 9 years before. Serum creatinine 2.1 mg/dl, creatinine clearance 27 ml/min, proteinuria 1.6 g/day. **a**, **b** Kidneys are reduced in volume (longitudinal diameter 8.4 and 8.5 cm), unstructured, with irregular profiles and hyperechoic parenchyma. **c** Intraparenchymal RIs are uniformly increased (0.72), except in the left mesorenal segment where the presence of a scar (**d**) is associated with RI of 0.83. L∅ = Longitudinal diameter.

When vasculitis determines advanced CKD stages, kidneys show non-specific signs: they can appear normal or reduced with a diffuse hyperechoic aspect (fig. 6). As in all forms of vasculitis, the anatomical damage affects not only glomerular capillaries but also renal microcirculation with deposition of complement and immunoglobulins thrombi. This justifies the widespread and marked RIs values during the acute phase (>0.75–0.80). In the chronic phase, RIs are typically >0.70.

Conclusion

Disreactive immunological disorders or non-inflammatory glomerular damage lead to secondary nephropathies. At US kidneys may appear normal or increased in volume in the early stages of disease and renal cortex may be hyperechoic if cell infiltration prevails or diffusely hypoechoic if edema prevails. RIs can be either high since the first stages of the disease (e.g., in amyloidosis, vasculitis) or they can increase as renal function impairs (e.g., in SLE). In any case, evaluation of renal morphology at B-mode US and vascular conditions at CD may be useful in first level diagnosis and in clinical follow-up of secondary chronic parenchymal diseases if they are associated with clinical patient history and biochemical parameters.

References

1 Stanley JH, Cornella R, Loevinger E, Schabel SI, Curry NS: Sonography of systemic lupus nephritis. AJR Am J Roentgenol 1984;142:1165–1168.
2 Platt JF, Rubin JM, Ellis JH: Lupus nephritis: predictive value of conventional and Doppler US and comparison with serologic and biopsy parameters. Radiology 1997;203:82–86.
3 D'Agati V, Appel GB: HIV infection and the kidney. J Am Soc Nephrol 1997;8:138–152.
4 Kay CJ: Renal diseases in patients with AIDS: sonographic findings. AJR Am J Roentgenol 1992;159:551–554.
5 Di Fiori JL, Rodrigue D, Kaptein EM, Ralls PW: Diagnostic sonography of HIV-associated nephropathy: new observations and clinical correlation. AJR Am J Roentgenol 1998;171:713–716.
6 Symeonidou C, Standish R, Sahdev A, Katz RD, Morlese J, Malhotra A: Imaging and histopathologic features of HIV-related renal disease. Radiographics 2008;28:1339–1354.
7 Atta MG, Longenecker JC, Fine DM, et al: Sonography as a predictor of human immunodeficiency virus-associated nephropathy. J Ultrasound Med 2004;23:603–610; quiz 612–613.
8 Wachsberg RH, Obolevich AT, Lasker N: Pelvocalyceal thickening in HIV-associated nephropathy. Abdom Imaging 1995;20:371–375.
9 Schaffer RM, Schwartz GE, Becker JA, Rao TK, Shih YH: Renal ultrasound in acquired immune deficiency syndrome. Radiology 1984;153:511–513.
10 Picken MM: Amyloidosis – where are we now and where are we heading? Arch Pathol Lab Med 2010;134:545–551.
11 West S, Singleton JD: Rheumatology Secrets, ed 2: Philadelphia, Hanley and Belfus, 2003.
12 Da'as N, Polliack A, Cohen Y, et al: Kidney involvement and renal manifestations in non-Hodgkin's lymphoma and lymphocytic leukemia: a retrospective study in 700 patients. Eur J Haematol 2001;67:158–164.
13 O'Riordan E, Reeve R, Houghton JB, O'Donoghue DJ, Waldek S: Primary bilateral T-cell renal lymphoma presenting with sudden loss of renal function. Nephrol Dial Transplant 2001;16:1487–1489.
14 Sheth S, Ali S, Fishman E: Imaging of renal lymphoma: patterns of disease with pathologic correlation. Radiographics 2006;26:1151–1168.
15 Dimopoulos MA, Kastritis E, Rosinol L, Bladé J, Ludwig H: Pathogenesis and treatment of renal failure in multiple myeloma. Leukemia 2008;22:1485–1493.
16 Hall MN, Jagannathan JP, Ramaiya NH, Shinagare AB, Van den Abbeele AD: Imaging of extraosseous myeloma: CT, PET/CT, and MRI features. AJR Am J Roentgenol 2010;195:1057–1065.
17 Savage CO: ANCA-associated renal vasculitis. Kidney Int 2001;60:1614–1627.

Mario Meola, MD, PhD
Department of Internal Medicine
Sant'Anna School of Advanced Studies, University of Pisa
Via Savi 10, IT–56126 Pisa (Italy)
E-Mail mario.meola@unipi.it; m.meola@sssup.it

Meola M, Petrucci I, Ronco C (eds): Ultrasound Imaging in Acute and Chronic Kidney Disease.
Contrib Nephrol. Basel, Karger, 2016, vol 188, pp 108–119 (DOI: 10.1159/000445473)

Clinical Scenarios in Chronic Kidney Disease: Chronic Tubulointerstitial Diseases

Mario Meola[a, b] • Sara Samoni[a, c] • Ilaria Petrucci[a, b]

[a]Sant'Anna School of Advanced Studies, Pisa, [b]Department of Internal Medicine, University of Pisa, Pisa, and [c]Department of Nephrology Dialysis and Transplantation, International Renal Research Institute (IRRIV), San Bortolo Hospital, Vicenza, Italy

Abstract

Chronic tubulointerstitial diseases are a common final pathway toward chronic renal failure regardless the primary damage (glomerular, vascular or directly the tubulointerstitium). Chronic tubulointerstitial nephritis (CTN) is characterized by interstitial scarring, fibrosis and tubule atrophy, resulting in progressive chronic kidney disease. Most frequent causes of CTN are drugs, heavy metals, obstructive uropathy, nephrolithiasis, reflux disease, immunologic diseases, neoplasia, ischemia, metabolic diseases, genetics and miscellaneous. At ultrasound (US), kidneys' morphological aspect is similar in all forms of chronic interstitial nephropathy and only chronic pyelonephritis with or without reflux shows distinguishing characteristics. In interstitial nephropathy, kidneys' profiles are finely irregular and corticomedullary differentiation is altered because of a diffused hyperechogenicity. The only indirect sign of chronic interstitial damage can be derived from the value of intrarenal resistive indexes that hardly overcome 0.75. US is mandatory in clinical chronic pyelonephritis work-up because it provides information on kidney's diameter and on growth nomogram in children. Renal profiles can be more or less altered depending on the number of cortical scars and the presence of pseudonodular areas of segmental compensatory hypertrophy. In the early stages, US diagnosis of renal tuberculosis is difficult because parenchymal lesions are non-specific. US sensitivity in the diagnosis of hydronephrosis is very high, close to 100% and, finally, US is the first choice imaging technique in the diagnosis of urinary lithiasis.

Chronic Tubulointerstitial Nephritis

Drug reactions (71–92% of cases) and infections are the most common causes of chronic tubulointerstitial nephritis (CTN). Anatomical damage is similar regardless the cause of interstitial damage. The most important histologic signs are interstitial fibrosis, lympho-monocyte's infiltration, tubules dilation with cell atrophy and basement membrane thickening. During the acute phase, glomeruli are not involved but in chronic damage a periglomerular fibrosis leading to segmental sclerosis and scleroatrophy is present. Instead, small arteries and arterioles show a different degree of fibrointimal thickening. Therefore, edema and lympho-monocyte's infiltration characterize acute interstitial nephropathy while fibrosis and tubular damage are the hallmarks of chronic interstitial damage. Clinical manifestations of renal damage (fall of glomerular filtration rate [GFR], mild proteinuria, hematuria, proximal or distal tubular acidosis, urine concentration disorders, mild hyperuricemia, anemia, high blood pressure) are associated with symptoms related to primary disease. In a series of patients with CTN, at the time of diagnosis creatinine clearance was <50 ml/min in 75% of cases and <15 ml/min in 33% of cases [1]. This means that in most cases, patients are referred to nephrologist and undergo ultrasound (US) examination when kidneys are already reduced in volume and diffusely hyperechoic.

As in all other causes of chronic kidney disease (CKD), the role of US varies depending on clinical context in this case also. US is commonly required to complete histological diagnosis performed during the acute phase of a chronic disease or to assess renal morphology of an unknown chronic disease in which clinical history and biochemical parameters suggest CTN. Kidneys' morphological aspect is similar in all forms of CTN and only chronic pyelonephritis with or without reflux shows distinguishing characteristics. In interstitial nephropathy, kidneys' profiles are finely irregular and corticomedullary differentiation is altered because of a diffused hyperechogenicity. These structural aspects are non-specific and do not allow to distinguish between interstitial chronic nephropathy due to analgesic abuse and any primitive or secondary interstitial damage (sarcoidosis, multiple myeloma, uric acid, lead, cadmium, lithium or hypopotassemia). US diagnosis of interstitial damage becomes even more difficult if kidneys' morphological analysis is performed by a non-nephrologist with little knowledge in clinical and laboratory data. In this case, the only US parameters that are routinely evaluated, that is, kidney volume, cortical and medullar echogenicity and urinary tract status, will lead to a non-specific report. The only indirect sign of chronic interstitial damage can be derived from the value of intrarenal resistive indexes (RIs) that hardly overcome 0.75.

Analgesic nephropathy is the most common cause of CTN, especially in women with a history of dysmenorrhea, headache and non-specific joint pain who routinely use non-steroidal anti-inflammatory drugs. It is mandatory to diagnose this form of CKD, because the progression of CKD to end-stage renal disease (ESRD) slows or stops if drug administration is interrupted. Patients with analgesic nephropathy are often referred to nephrologist because of nocturia, hypertension and fall of GFR. It is very common to find also urothelial tumors. Histological damage is non-specific and shows the typical features of a chronic interstitial nephritis, sometimes associated with papillary necrosis. At US, kidneys show a reduced volume, with irregular profiles and lost corticomedullary differentiation. Commonly, both kidneys show a diffuse hyperechoic aspect that affects cortex and renal pyramids. Hyperechoic plaques secondary to fibrosis and microcalcifications at the apex of renal papillae can be very useful to diagnose tubulointerstitial damage secondary to analgesics. Papillary necrosis is more evident with contrast-enhanced CT, although this technique is contraindicated in patients with impaired renal function [2]. Endemic Balkan nephropathy is a CTN of Balkan areas with an unknown etiology. Calcium metabolism disturbances and, more rarely, the presence of granulomatous lesions are responsible of tubulointerstitial damage in sarcoidosis nephropathy. A total of 10–15% of patients with sarcoidosis show, in fact, hypercalcemic hypercalciuria that determines tubular disorders, reduces GFR and favors nephrocalcinosis or kidney stones. US signs of nephrocalcinosis and/or kidney stones get overlapped with non-specific signs of interstitial involvement.

Chronic interstitial damage in myeloma may be due to clogging of renal tubular lumens with plugs (casts) containing 'light chains' ('cast nephropathy') or to hypercalcemia, nephrocalcinosis and/or hyperuricemia. Kidneys' aspect varies depending on which factor has determined renal damage. In cast nephropathy, kidneys are hypoechoic, with normal or increased volume, depending on edema and tubular damage. When glomerular deposition of amyloid prevails, kidneys appear normal or increased in volume and diffusely hyperechoic, while in hypercalcemic and/or hyperuricemic chronic forms, cortex is diffusely hyperechoic and medulla can be either hyperechoic (due to uric acid or calcium salts deposition), or hypoechoic with a hyperechoic edge due to nephrocalcinosis. Tumor lysis syndrome is a known cause of acute kidney injury (AKI), because it determines severe hyperuricemia. On the contrary, not all authors agree to consider this disorder as a cause of chronic interstitial disease (gouty nephropathy or chronic uric acid nephropathy) (fig. 1).

Chronic interstitial uric acid deposition accelerates kidney damage but at US it does not show characteristic morphological signs. Even chronic inherited or acquired hypokalemia can cause chronic interstitial nephropathy. Hypokalemic

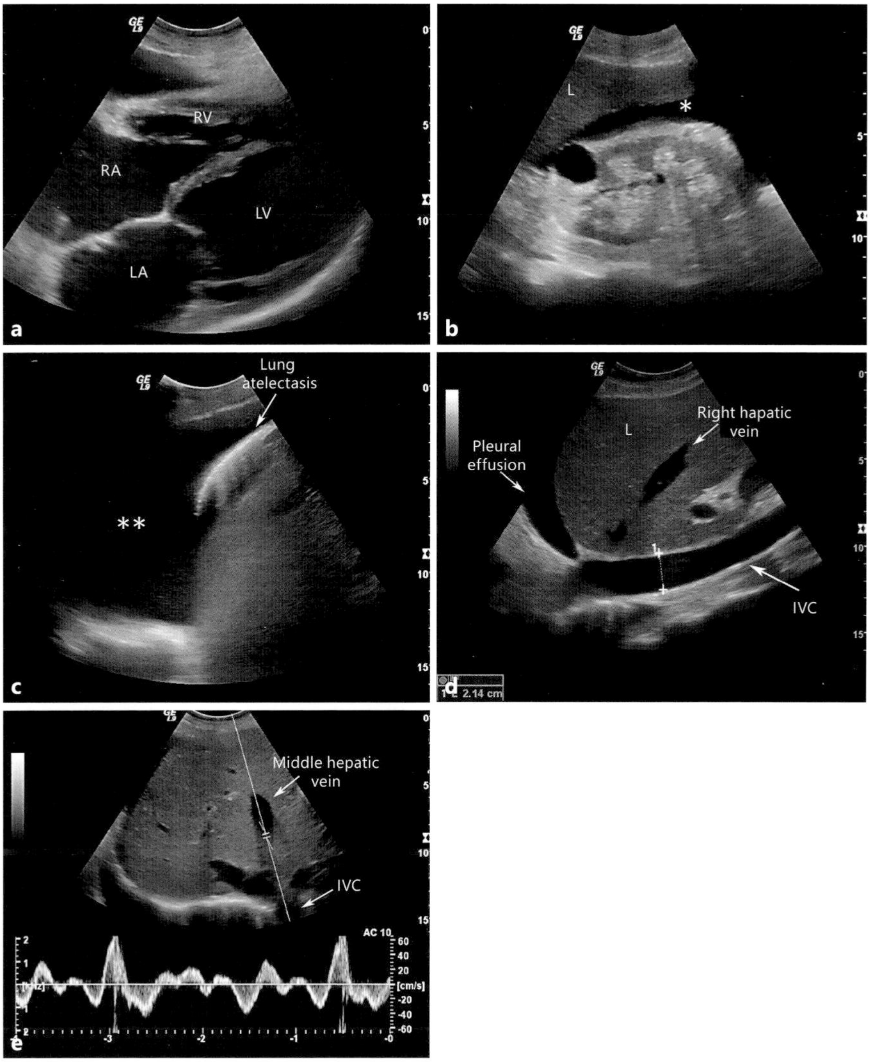

Fig. 1. Uric acid nephropathy associated with cardio renal syndrome type 2. Male, aged 57 years, with biventricular failure of previous anterior STEMI. Clinical history of gout, hyperuricemia and uric acid lithiasis. Serum creatinine 3.4 mg/dl, GFR 22 ml/min. **a** Cardiorenal syndrome type 2: post-infarction dilated cardiomyopathy with signs of right overload. **b** Both kidneys are reduced in volume (longitudinal diameter 9 cm) with reduced cortical thickness, hyperechoic pyramids and few acquired cysts. Right kidney pyramids show a nephrocalcinosis secondary to hyperuricuria. Ascites (*) and pleural effusion (**) (**c**). **d** Dilated and rigid Inferior Vena Cava (white arrows). **e** Central suprahepatic vein overload. RA = Right atrium; RV = right ventricle; LA = left atrium; LV = left ventricle; L = liver; IVC = inferior vena cava.

nephropathy is characterized by renal loss of potassium, normal blood pressure and high urinary excretion of renin, aldosterone and prostaglandin E. At US, kidneys show a widespread hyperechogenicity of cortex and renal pyramids edges, as in early nephrocalcinosis. US features do not have a clear correspondence with histological damage, characterized by the presence of vacuoles with undefined content in proximal convoluted tubule cells. Hyperoxaluria may be either inherited or acquired. Intratubular precipitation of calcium oxalate causes fibrosis, tubular atrophy and kidney function impairment. At US, kidneys with oxalosis are reduced in volume with a thin corticomedullary thickness. Loss of parenchymal differentiation and high cortical and medullar hyperechogenicity are determined by fibrosis and nephrocalcinosis. Hyperechoic microspots and microaggregates along the corticomedullary junction and medulla are very common structural aspects [3].

Lead nephropathy is an occupational disease caused by prolonged lead exposure. Proximal tubular cells of renal tubules absorb lead. In children, lead causes interstitial nephropathy with isolated tubular defects or Fanconi syndrome. In adults, however, lead causes CKD with interstitial fibrosis, tubular atrophy and nephrosclerosis associated with hyperuricemia, gout and high blood pressure (fig. 2). The lack of a sensitive and specific diagnostic test, except the lead urine dosage after 2 doses of EDTA (ethylene diamine tetra-acetic acid) justifies the common delay in diagnosis. At US, kidneys' aspect is non-specific as in cadmium nephropathy, an occupational disease of foundry workers, or in lithium and mercury nephropathy. Radiation nephropathy is a chronic interstitial nephropathy that sub-clinically manifests with GFR reduction, severe hypertension and mild proteinuria in patients undergoing radiotherapy >23 gray without protective screens. Sonographic appearance of fibrotic kidneys is amorphous, although sometimes it can be associated with mild urinary tract dilation, secondary to retroperitoneal actinic fibrosis.

Kidney with chronic pyelonephritis shows more specific characteristics than that of chronic interstitial nephropathy. The prevalence of chronic pyelonephritis is not well known. In the USA transplants register, the frequency of chronic pyelonephritis as a cause of ESRD is 13%. Parenchymal scar is the primary lesion of chronic pyelonephritis, that is, an irregular retraction of kidney profile that may or may not be associated with dilation, deformity and corticalization of calyces below (fig. 3). Only vesicoureteral reflux (VUR), obstructive uropathy, papillary necrosis secondary to analgesics or atypical papillary necrosis due to dehydration or sickle cell disease can lead to a morphological feature similar to pyelonephritic kidney. Only in a small number of patients, cortical scars and calyceal deformities may be evident even in the absence of such conditions or without any bacterial infection. Therefore, chronic pyelonephritis can be divid-

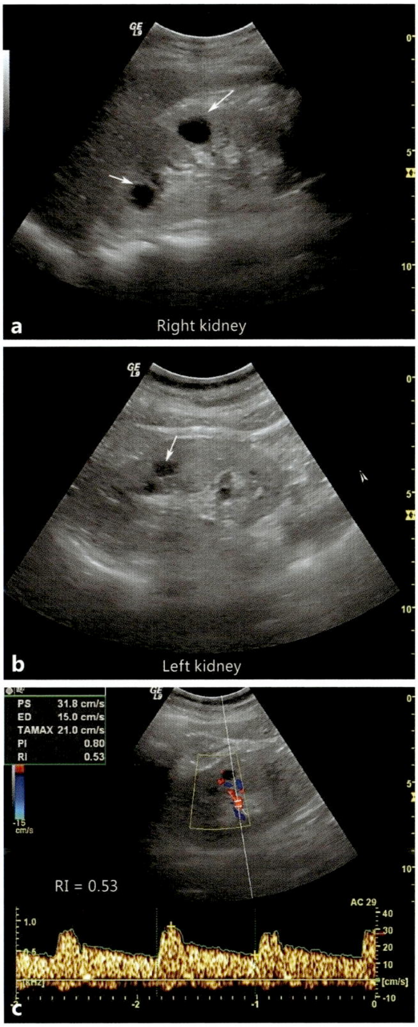

Fig. 2. Chronic Lead Tubulointerstitial Nephropathy. Male, aged 29 years, with neurosensory hypoacusis, cardiac and muscle glycogenose and stage 3 CKD associated with proteinuria <1 g/day. Histological diagnosis of focal segmental glomerulonephritis and lead poisoning at the age of 23. **a**, **b** Kidneys are well shaped and have normal profiles. Coronal diameter is 9.5–10 cm. Parenchymal structure is altered and hyperechoic with multiple acquired cysts (white arrows). No evidence of papillary or pyramidal calcifications. The morphological aspect is compatible with a chronic interstitial nephropathy but RIs are very low (0.53) (**c**).

ed into 3 types: (1) chronic pyelonephritis with reflux (reflux nephropathy), (2) chronic pyelonephritis with obstruction (obstructive nephropathy) and (3) chronic idiopathic pyelonephritis.

US is mandatory in clinical chronic pyelonephritis work-up because it provides information on kidney's diameter and on growth nomogram in children. Renal profiles can be more or less altered depending on the number of cortical scars (triangular hyperechoic areas) and the presence of pseudonodular areas of segmental compensatory hypertrophy [4]. Pseudo-nodular parenchyma looks like a pseudomass; so differential diagnosis with contrast-enhanced US (CEUS) is needed to exclude the presence of a tumor. Scars are poorly or non-vascular-

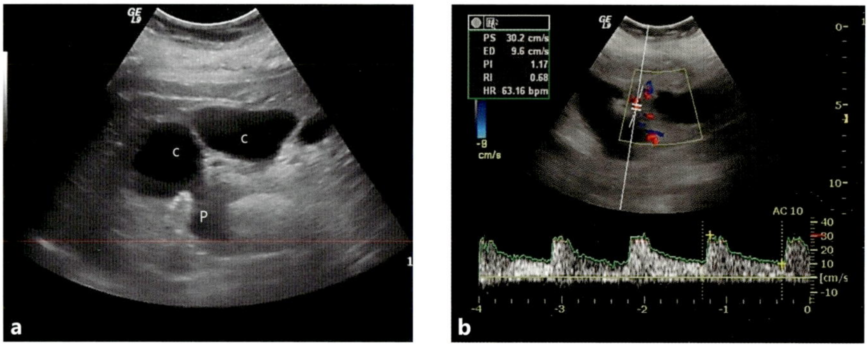

Fig. 3. Chronic reflux pyelonephritis. Female, aged 58 years. Serum creatinine 1.3 mg/dl, GFR 48 ml/min. Cystourethroplasty at the age of 30 years. **a** Left renal parenchyma disruption with scars and corticalization of medial and inferior calyces. **b** Upper pole residual parenchyma with RI of 0.68. P = Pelvis; c = calyces.

ized, and RIs are high. On the contrary, in hypertrophic areas, renal vessels show the normal radial distribution and RIs are normal or slightly elevated. In end stage, pyelonephritic kidney is small, shrunk and shows a hyperechoic unstructured parenchyma; so it becomes impossible to distinguish the renal sinus from the parenchyma.

Post-primary tuberculosis (TB) mainly affects lungs and genitourinary tract. Renal parenchyma, urinary tract (ureter and bladder) and genital system (testis, seminal tract) are renal TB targets. Cortical tubercle is the primary lesion of urogenital tuberculosis, due to blood borne infection. The miliary tubercles formed subsequent to blood borne infection begin to spread, resulting in caseous cavitary necrosis. Necrotic caseous material is released into the medulla, thus generating cold abscesses that join the papillo-calyceal junction. Debris containing tubercle bacilli are consequently discharged into the ureter; so inflammatory process ends but fibrosis and calyceal stenosis/amputation become prevalent. Mastic kidney shows parenchymal cavitations mixed with calcifications and fibrosis areas [5]. In the early stages, US diagnosis of renal TB is difficult because parenchymal lesions are non-specific. Cavitations appear as confluent and irregular cystic-like lesions, closed or opened into the urinary tract (calyces, pelvis). In these cases, urinary tract is hypotonic and dilated and shows a thickened urothelium, sometimes with calcifications. These structural aspects need a differential diagnosis with urothelioma or other infectious forms. Normally, opened tubercular cavitations are associated with multiple calcifications and irregular parenchymal scars that alter kidney's profile. Sometimes, kidney shows only non-specific signs. In these cases, diagnosis of urinary TB is suggested by ureter hypotonia associated with microbladder in a patient with a non-specific urinary tract infection with fever and acid pyuria. Less frequently, TB is diagnosed after the evidence of complex lesions affecting testis, epididymis and vas deferens. Mastic kidney does not show a different aspect from pyelonephritic or a xanthogranulomatous kidney and diagnosis must be confirmed with CT or MRI [6].

Non-Inflammatory Tubulointerstitial Diseases

Reflux Nephropathy

The term 'reflux nephropathy' highlights the primary role of VUR in the pathogenesis of chronic pyelonephritis. In 1981, the International Reflux Study Committee proposed a 5 grades classification of VUR [7]. In VUR grade I, voiding cystography (or cystoscintigraphy/cystography with CEUS) shows a post-void reflux in the lumbar ureter. In VUR grade II reflux interests all the pyelocaliceal system, with no dilation. In VUR grade III and IV, pyelocaliceal and ureteral dilation appears and worsens. In these stages, calyces are corticalized, parenchymal thickness is reduced and renal profiles are altered. In severe and chronic grade V reflux, imaging techniques show corticalization of calyces with an important reduction of parenchymal thickness. Globular pelvis is followed by a dilated and tortuous ureter, while calyces show thickened walls and a clubbed morphology (fig. 4) [8]. In younger patients, urinary infections are the most common complication of reflux and cause a progressive loss of GFR until ESRD.

Obstructive Nephropathy

CKD secondary to obstruction is called chronic obstructive nephropathy. Stenosis may involve the pelvis (ureteropelvic junction stenosis, lithiasis, tumors), the ureter (lithiasis, tumors, ab extrinseco compression) or the lower urinary tract (bladder, prostate and urethra). Urine flow is hindered by mechanical obstruction, thus leading to a progressive renal damage also due to increased hydrostatic pressure in the urinary tract. Kidney shows a gross dilation/ballooning of the renal pelvis in severe hydronephrosis with a complete parenchymal loss. Severe hydronephrosis can affect only intrarenal calyces and pelvis or may extend to the ureter with a coexistent bladder stasis in case of a lower urinary tract stenosis. In severe hydronephrosis, renal pelvis is anechoic and calyces appear dilated, clubbed, anechoic and corticalized, while the ureter is dilated and tortuous along its whole length. US sensitivity in the diagnosis of hydronephrosis is very high, close to 100% [9]. In hydropyonephrosis, pyelocaliceal cavities are heterogeneous due to the presence of purulent corpuscular material, mixed with

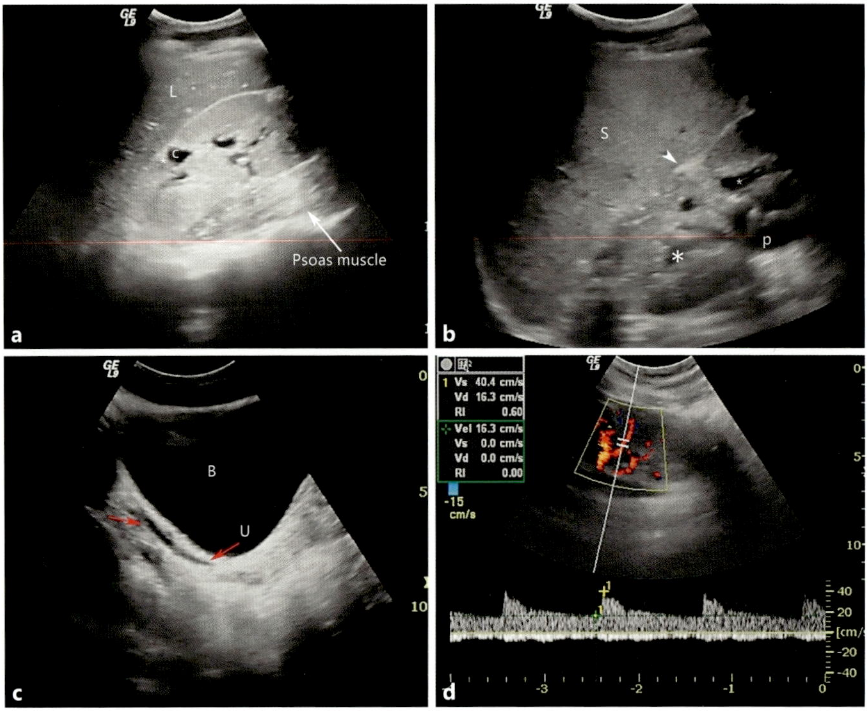

Fig. 4. Chronic reflux nephropathy. Bilateral VUR treated with cystourethroplasty. **a**, **b** Kidneys show segmental scars (arrowhead) with corticalization of calyces and mild dilation of the excretory system (*). Normal parenchymal segments appear hyperechoic. **c** Distended bladder shows regular walls. Ureteral opening is normal but the pre-mural tract and pelvic ureter are dilated (red arrow). **d** Intraparenchymal RIs are not increased. L = Liver; S = spleen; p = pelvis; B = bladder; U = ureter; c = calyx.

hyperechoic bridles. Typically, hydropyonephrosis may be associated with struvite stones or with xanthogranulomatous pyelonephritis.

US is the first choice imaging technique in the diagnosis of urinary lithiasis [10]. At B-Mode imaging, calcium, uric acid or cystine stones appear as hyperechoic concretions located in the urinary tract with a posterior acoustic shadowing. The posterior acoustic shadowing is a useful artifact, and if it is present in all scans, it represents a sure sign of lithiasis. Struvite calculi represent 15–20% of kidney stones. Struvite calculi are commonly staghorn and they reproduce the pelvis and urinary tract form (fig. 5). For this reason, US is not able to characterize the entire calculus but it shows only the presence of hyperechoic separate fragments into the pelvis and in the major and minor papillae. Staghorn calculi are frequently associated with simple or infected hydronephrosis. Calculi can be formed more rarely in the lumen of calyceal diverticula or into an ureterocele. Benign prostatic hyperplasia can cause bladder stones in men.

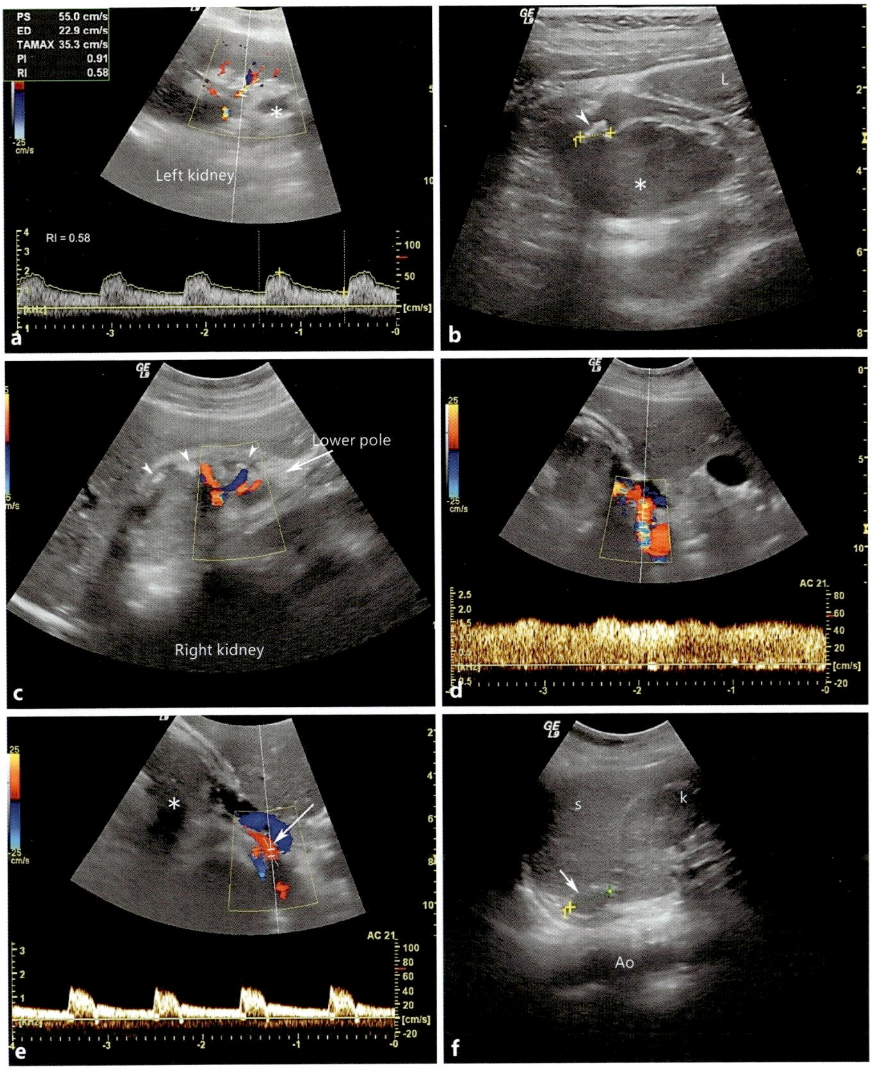

Fig. 5. Chronic obstructive nephropathy secondary to lithiasis. Chronic obstructive nephropathy of the right kidney due to staghorn lithiasis treated with laparoscopic litholapaxy. Acute post-treatment hematoma with acute renal failure. **a** Left kidney with pyelic hypotonia (*). **b** Right kidney is disrupted with reduced parenchymal thickness. Iatrogenic parenchymal hematoma appears as a pseudo-nodular hypoechoic mass (*), not vascularized, that occupies the entire renal sinus. Multiple lithiasis (arrowhead). **c** Color Doppler shows a small amount of vascularized parenchyma in the inferior polar region. The hypotonic urinary tract is difficult to recognize with US and contains stones of 7 and 9 mm (arrowhead). **d** Right renal vein and (**e**) artery are well perfused. **f** Small incidentaloma of the right adrenal gland (white arrow). L = Liver; S = spleen; Ao = aorta; R = right kidney; k = kidney.

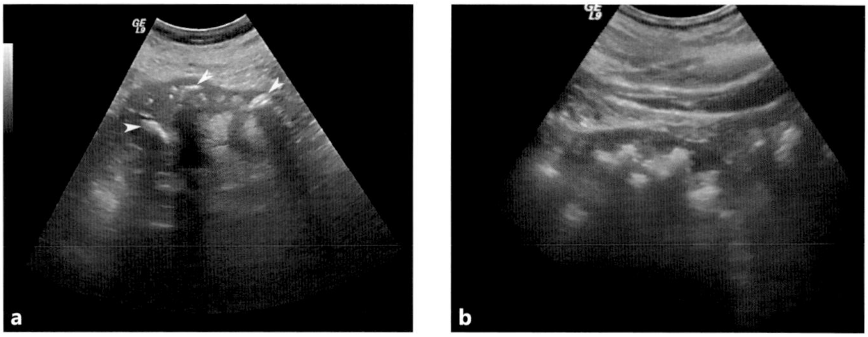

Fig. 6. Chronic obstructive nephropathy secondary to lithiasis. In end-stage CKD, the presence of staghorn (**a**), cystine (**b**) or other type of lithiasis may or may not be associated with hydronephrosis. In reported cases, the kidney is reduced in volume, unstructured, with multiple lithiasis (arrowhead) in the non-dilated urinary tract.

As the prostate enlarges, it can compress the urethra and interrupt urine flow, causing urine to remain in the bladder. Also bladder muscle disorders (paraplegia, neurogenic bladder) or chronic immobilization can cause bladder stones. Actually, US multifrequency probes have a spatial resolution that can detect calculi with diameter >4.5 mm. Smaller calculi generate hyperechoic spots without posterior acoustic shadowing. Color Doppler confirms the calcific component of calculi showing the 'twinkling artifact' [11]. Therefore, it is a conceptual mistake to report the term 'kidney sand' in the diagnostic conclusions. Calculi in major and minor calyces can be easily localized, even when calculi are small. The diagnosis in these cases is easier if lithiasis is associated with hydrocalyces, while it becomes difficult in the absence of dilation of the urinary tract, if the calculus is in the pelvis or it has been moved into the ureter after a reno-ureteral colic. In fact, US sensitivity in the diagnosis of renal lithiasis is very high (95%), while in ureteral lithiasis is reduced to 30–35% [12, 13]. If pyelectasis is absent, pelvic small calculi can be movable or masked by sinus hyperechogenicity. Acoustic posterior shadowing can be masked by multiple sinus interfaces or by the air into the colic flexure. Colic air can also mask solitary ureteral calculus stone fragments after extracorporeal shock wave lithotripsy (stein-Strasse). Ureteral calculi blocked into the ureterovesical junction are well evident. So, the ureter segment between iliac vessels and ureterovesical junction is the most difficult part to study with US. In chronic obstructive disease secondary to lithiasis, kidney is reduced in volume and parenchymal thickness becomes progressively thinner and disrupted. In end stages, obstruction may be associated or not with hydronephrosis, despite the origin of calculi (fig. 6).

Conclusion

At US, kidneys' morphological aspect is similar in all forms of chronic interstitial nephropathy and only chronic pyelonephritis with or without reflux shows distinguishing characteristics. In interstitial nephropathy, kidney profiles are finely irregular and corticomedullary differentiation is diffusely hyperechoic. The only indirect sign of chronic interstitial damage is that RI hardly overcomes 0.75. In early stages, US diagnosis of renal tuberculosis is difficult because parenchymal lesions are non-specific. US sensitivity in hydronephrosis is close to 100% and, finally, US is the first choice imaging technique in the diagnosis of urinary lithiasis.

References

1 Eknoyan G, McDonald MA, Appel D, Truong LD: Chronic tubulo-interstitial nephritis: correlation between structural and functional findings. Kidney Int 1990;38:736–743.
2 Elseviers MM, De schepper A, Corthouts R, et al: High diagnostic performance of CT scan for analgesic nephropathy in patients with incipient to severe renal failure. Kidney Int 1995;48:1316–1323.
3 Kraus RA, Gaisie G, Young LW: Increased renal parenchymal echogenicity: causes in pediatric patients. Radiographics 1990;10: 1009–1018.
4 Puech P, Lagard D, Leroy C, Dracon M, Biserte J, Lemaître L: [Imaging in urinary tract infections in adults]. J Radiol 2004;85(2 pt 2):220–240.
5 Becker JA: Renal tuberculosis. Urol Radiol 1988;10:25–30.
6 Rui X, Li XD, Cai S, et al: Ultrasonographic diagnosis and typing of renal tuberculosis. Int J Urol 2008;15:135–139.
7 Medical versus surgical treatment of primary vesicoureteral reflux: a prospective international reflux study in children. J Urol 1981; 125:277–283.
8 Bailey RR, Lynn KL: End-stage reflux nephropathy. Contrib Nephrol 1984;39:102–110.
9 Talner Lb,O'reilly Ph, Roy C, et al: Urinary obstruction; in Pollack HM, McClennan BL (eds): Clinical Uropathy, ed 2. Philadelphia, WB Saunders, 2000, vol 2, pp 1846–1966.
10 Riccabona M, Fotter R: Urinary tract infection in infants and children: an update with special regard to the changing role of reflux. Eur Radiol 2004;14(suppl 4):L78–L88.
11 Kamaya A, Tuthill T, Rubin JM: Twinkling artifact on color Doppler sonography: dependence on machine parameters and underlying cause. AJR Am J Roentgenol 2003;180: 215–222.
12 Bush WH, Cho JY, Chung JW, et al: Urolithiasis, Elsevier Science, 2003, pp 371–373.
13 Kameda T, Kawai F, Taniguchi N, et al: Ultrasonography for ureteral stone detection in patients with or without caliceal dilatation. J Med Ultrasonics 2010;37:9–14.

Mario Meola, MD, PhD
Department of Internal Medicine
Sant'Anna School of Advanced Studies, University of Pisa
Via Savi 10, IT–56126 Pisa (Italy)
E-Mail mario.meola@unipi.it; m.meola@sssup.it

Meola M, Petrucci I, Ronco C (eds): Ultrasound Imaging in Acute and Chronic Kidney Disease.
Contrib Nephrol. Basel, Karger, 2016, vol 188, pp 120–130 (DOI: 10.1159/000445474)

Clinical Scenarios in Chronic Kidney Disease: Cystic Renal Diseases

Mario Meola[a, b] • Sara Samoni[a, c] • Ilaria Petrucci[a, b]

[a]Sant'Anna School of Advanced Studies, Pisa, [b]Department of Internal Medicine, University of Pisa, Pisa, and [c]Department of Nephrology Dialysis and Transplantation, International Renal Research Institute (IRRIV), San Bortolo Hospital, Vicenza, Italy

Abstract

Cysts are frequently found in chronic kidney disease (CKD) and they have a different prognostic significance depending on the clinical context. Simple solitary parenchymal cysts and peripelvic cysts are very common and they have no clinical significance. At US, simple cyst appears as a round anechoic pouch with regular and thin profiles. On the other hand, hereditary polycystic disease is a frequent cause of CKD in children and adults. Autosomal dominant polycystic kidney disease (ADPKD) and autosomal recessive polycystic kidney disease (ARPKD) are the best known cystic hereditary diseases. ADPKD and ARPKD show a diffused cystic degeneration with cysts of different diameters derived from tubular epithelium. Medullary cystic disease may be associated with tubular defects, acidosis and lithiasis and can lead to CKD. Acquired cystic kidney disease, finally, is secondary to progressive structural end-stage kidney remodelling and may be associated with renal cell carcinoma.

Introduction

All cystic kidney diseases have a primary benign lesion in common – the cyst – which is a serous fluid-filled sac (fig. 1). The pathogenesis of simple cysts is unknown. On the contrary, hereditary and congenital cysts pathogenesis is due to gene mutations that alter the function of proteins needed for the integrity of tubular epithelium primary cilia [1, 2].

Ultrasound (US) imaging is very sensitive and specific in the diagnosis of kidney cysts (fig. 1) and it is pivotal in the active surveillance of complex cysts and inherited/congenital diseases.

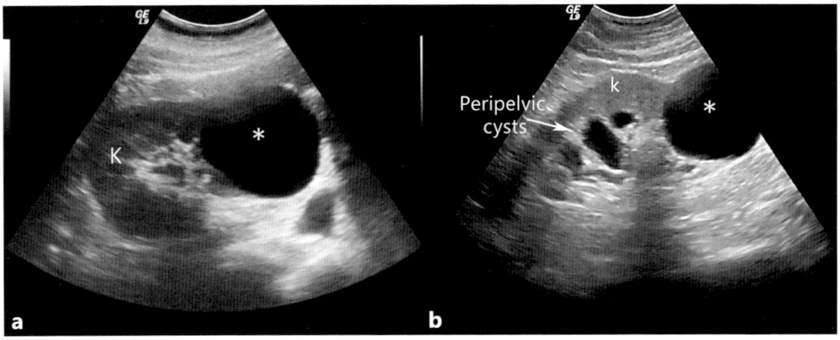

Fig. 1. Renal simple cyst. Simple parenchymal cyst is an expansive round lesion, a serous fluid-filled sac. It may grow in the parenchyma or toward the extrarenal space. Cystic liquid is limpid, citrine and a layer of fibrous connective tissue coated on the luminal side by a thin layer of thin and regular epithelial cells constitutes the walls. **a** Transverse scans on right kidney hilum. Simple cysts with smooth walls and anechoic content (*). Slight rain artifact of the near wall. Posterior acoustic enhancement has been smoothed to show the inferior vena cava. The lateral acoustic cone is accentuated by the relationships between cystic convex surface and right colon content. **b** Coronal scan of left kidney. Simple parenchymal exophytic cyst of the lower pole (*) and small peripelvic cyst (arrow). K and k = Kidney.

Simple and Peripelvic Cysts

At US, simple cyst appears as a round anechoic pouch with regular and thin profiles. Fluid content and curved profiles generate 2 useful artifacts for differential diagnosis of cysts (fig. 1): (1) the posterior acoustic enhancement on the distal wall, which is generated by reflection of the slightly attenuated US beam and (2) the lateral acoustic cones resulting from the attenuation/refraction of incident US beam on the cyst convex edge.

Cyst wall remodelling secondary to bleeding or infection requires careful differential diagnosis with cystic renal cell carcinoma (RCC), which accounts for 10% of all kidney tumours. Bosniak classification of cysts, based on CT with contrast medium [3], states that simple cyst appears as a fluid-filled expansive lesion (Bosniak Class I) (fig. 2). Rarely the cyst has a complex structure, characterized by the presence of small and thin endocystic septa and/or non-enhanced microcalcifications (Bosniak Class II) (fig. 2).

At US, cysts in class I-II show the same structural characteristics, they are benign lesions and do not require active surveillance. When cyst wall or septa appear thicker and show irregular calcifications, the probability of a cystic carcinoma is near 50% of cases, in particular, if there is contrast medium enhancement (Bosniak Class III) (fig. 2).

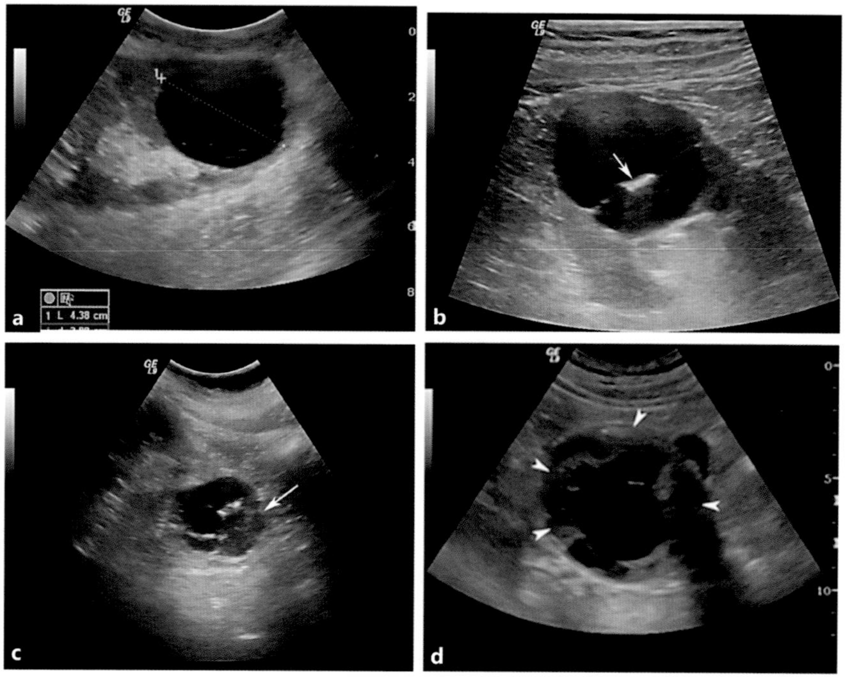

Fig. 2. Bosniak classification of cysts. **a** Class I renal cyst of the left renal pole. Class I cysts have thin and regular walls, without no septa, wall thickening or calcifications. At contrast-enhanced CT, they are not enhanced with contrast media. Class I cysts do not require monitoring or treatment. **b** Class II renal cyst with an intracystic septum and a small linear calcification. Class II cysts are benign, well defined, but they have some rare septa with thickness <1 mm or some linear calcifications. At CT, there is no enhancement of walls or septa. **c** Class IIF renal cyst. These cysts contain a greater number of thickened septa. Walls are thickened but regular, without enhancement. The image shows a complex cyst with multiple septa and structured content (arrow). **d** Class III cyst. Cysts have multiple thickened septa, wall plaques or nodules and multiple calcifications. The percentage of malignancy is ~54%. The image shows a complex cyst with thickened and irregular walls, hypo and hyperechoic tissue bridles, mixed with parietal calcification (arrowhead).

Cysts with a diameter >3 cm, especially if they show a hemorrhagic content and a structure classified Bosniak II or III, are grouped in class IIF (F = follow-up). In other words, these complex lesions need a 6-month/annual monitoring (fig. 2). If cystic wall or septa thickening show a solid or nodular appearance with irregular calcifications, this cyst is included in Bosniak Class IV because this complex lesion is almost a carcinoma. Second harmonic US imaging, spatial composite imaging and color Doppler have significantly improved the US sensitivity in the classification of cysts [4], although the differential diagnosis of complex cysts requires the use of contrast-enhanced US [5, 6].

Peripelvic cysts are lymphatic collections into the renal sinus (fig. 1). Sometimes, in children they may be associated with dilated intra- and perirenal lymphatic vessels, thus determining lymphangiectasia or parapelvic lymphangiomatosis [7]. Peripelvic cysts are common in adults and they are often multiple, bilateral and not confluent. Sometimes, a cluster of peripelvic cysts can occupy the entire renal sinus. They are almost asymptomatic but they can cause hematuria, compression/hydronephrosis and hypertension [8]. Differential diagnosis between hydronephrosis and peripelvic cysts is based on specific signs: (1) peripelvic cysts are not communicating lesions; (2) in hydronephrosis there is an evident communication between calyces, pelvis and ureter; (3) peripelvic cysts have irregular profiles and very variable size; (4) dilated calyces appear regular and rounded with an evident relationship with renal papilla which appears flattened [9].

Hereditary Cystic Diseases

Autosomal dominant polycystic kidney disease (ADPKD) and autosomal recessive polycystic kidney disease (ARPKD) are the best known cystic hereditary diseases. ADPKD and ARPKD show a diffuse cystic degeneration with cysts of different diameters derived from tubular epithelium. ADPKD is caused by mutations in *PKD1* and *PKD2* genes encoding PC-1 and PC-2 complex proteins, which are cilium and intercellular junction glycoproteins. All typical cases of ARPKD are due to mutations of the *PKHD1* gene in a single locus, coding for fibrocystin/polyductin. Inheritance modalities, clinical presentation and type of kidney damage reflect the different pathogenesis of ADPKD and ARPKD. Autosomal dominant medullary cystic kidney disease (ADMCKD) is a dominant hereditary tubulointerstitial disease caused by mutations in the gene encoding uromodulin or Tamm–Horsfall protein. Nephrocystin is a protein involved in the organization of apical junctions and in the control of epithelial cell polarity. Nephrocystin dysfunction due to an autosomal recessive defect leads to medullary nephronophthisis (NPH).

Polycystic Disease in Adults and Children

ADPKD is the most frequent hereditary cystic disease (5% of the dialysis population) and its clinical manifestations appear between 30 and 50 years [10]. All imaging techniques are sensitive in the diagnosis of ADPKD, but second level imaging also play a critical role in the evaluation of complications and of disease

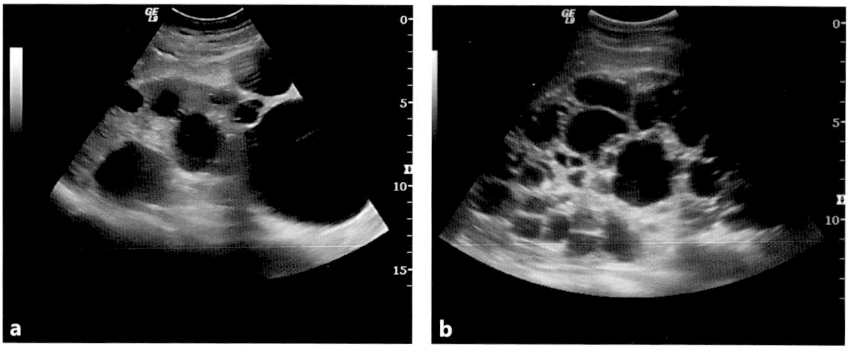

Fig. 3. ADPKD. **a** Early stages. The image shows cysts of different diameter with parenchymal thickness almost present. **b** In advanced stages, renal parenchyma is completely replaced by cysts that favour functional impairment due to obstructive and ischemic phenomena. Kidney volume is increased and cystic degeneration does not allow defining renal morphology as kidney occupies the left abdominal space until the pelvic cavity.

progression following medical treatments (e.g., sirolymus or vaptans). US is the first level imaging, but it is not very sensitive in measuring the coronal diameter of an increased kidney and in the identification of cysts ∅ <5 mm. Thus, US is not always able to reveal the first signs of a polycystic disease [11]. ADPKD diagnostic criteria are based on detection of cysts in one or both kidneys. In order to suspect ADPKD, there must be at least 2 cysts evident in each kidney if patient is aged between 30 and 59, and at least 4 cysts in each kidney after 60 years. [12].

Polycystic kidney structure varies according to the severity and stage of the disease (fig. 3). In the first stages, kidneys are increased in volume (longitudinal diameter >13 cm) and there is a widespread presence of cysts with different diameter in the medulla and cortex. Parenchyma between the cysts is hyperechoic and full of microspots due to reflection phenomenon of microscopic developing cysts. At colour Doppler, kidneys show a progressive microvascular rarefaction while larger vessels run in residual parenchyma septa. In early stages, resistive indexes (RIs) are not high due to the intra-renal blood flow redistribution. RIs are significantly increased only in end pre-dialytic stages and in dialysis patients. Cysts diameter and morphology vary depending on compression and involutive phenomena. Disease progression is more rapid when small diameter cysts (<3 cm) prevail, although severity of renal damage, as well as clinical manifestations, varies in the same family line and in different families.

Cystic bleeding is commonly accompanied by back pain (fig. 4) and sometimes by hematuria and clots. Back pain may be absent if bleeding is slight; so this complication is detected only by US which highlights a corpuscular and hyperechoic content in complicated cysts. If there is an important intracystic

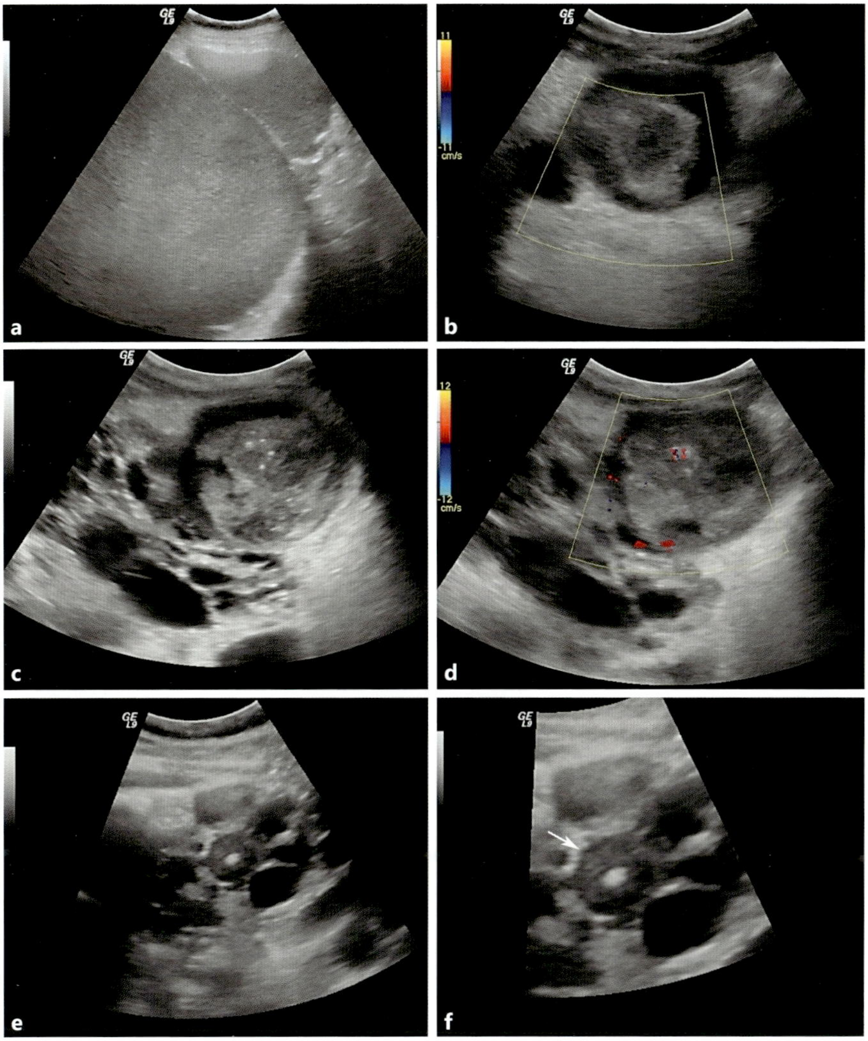

Fig. 4. ADPKD and intracystic bleeding. The sudden onset of lower back pain indicates that intracystic bleeding has caused a sudden distension of cystic walls. **a** Intracystic hemorrhage in patient treated with warfarin after cardiac valve replacement. Cyst diameter is >19 cm. **b** Cyst with clot with no signs of color Doppler perfusion. **c**, **d** Microcalcification in an organized clot with twinkling artifact. Absence of vascular perfusion. **e**, **f** Organized clot with calcified protein matrix (arrow) (small and high magnification).

bleeding, cysts volume quickly increases thus causing lower back pain. Intracystic blood forms a clot that generates intermediate level echoes, which can stratify until filling cystic cavitiy. Clot retraction makes the cyst become a complex mass with irregular vacuoles bounded by hyperechoic septa and bridles adherent to the wall and filled with corpuscular material and debris (fig. 4). Clot debris are absorbed very slowly so the cyst appears as a complex mass for several months. In these cases, a differential diagnosis between complex cyst and cystic carcinoma is needed. Unlike bleeding, cyst rupture is a very rare event [13].

Hypertension is present in 75% of cases, almost occurring before any significant reduction in renal function, with an average age onset of 30 years. Left ventricle hypertrophy tends to develop even earlier in patients with ADPKD and it is well evident in subxiphoid scans [14]. Abdominal aortic aneurysm is less frequent than cerebral aneurysm of Willis circle, which occurs in 4–10% of patients and undergoes rupture in 25% of cases [15]. Liver cysts of different diameter are very common (75% of cases) and they are widespread in both lobes. As renal cysts, they are silent but can become symptomatic for bleeding, rupture or infection. Sometimes, as a result of an excessive growth that compresses the diaphragm, they can cause dyspnea, orthopnea, early satiety, vomiting, rib fracture, uterine prolapse and abdominal hernias. If liver cysts compress biliary tract and portal and systemic venous vessels, they can cause jaundice, portal hypertension, hepatic/caval vein thrombosis or Budd Chiari syndrome. Lithiasis is a rare complication in ADPKD, which is induced by a reduced citrate excretion and cystic compression on the urinary tract [16].

ARPKD diagnosis is often prenatal. US with high-resolution probes shows an increased volume of fetal kidneys which appear hyperechoic, with multiple cortical and medullary microcysts and without corticomedullary differentiation [17]. Renal cortex, in particular, appears hyperechoic due to the high number of acoustic interfaces generated between microcysts around collecting tubules [17]. ARPKD differential diagnosis can be difficult if renal involvement is slight, because kidney size is normal and hyperechogenicity is not accompanied by the presence of cysts. During the pre- and perinatal period, cysts increase in number and size.

When hepatic fibrosis prevails, liver is increased in volume for widespread steatofibrosis associated with intrahepatic bile ducts dilation, as in bile duct atresia or Caroli's disease. Periportal fibrosis causes portal hypertension, reduced portal flow volume, portal vein and splenorenal/mesenteric axis ectasia, splenomegaly, splenic peri-hilar varicosity and antropyloric region wall thickening due to varicose veins. Few studies have evaluated the long-term follow-up of ARPKD due to the low survival of these patients, but they show that liver parenchyma echogenicity remains stable and cysts number does not grow [18]. In late referral with hepatic failure and portal hypertension, kidneys may be normal or enlarged because of bilateral multiple cysts that simulate ADPKD. In these patients, a liver biopsy is needed for differential diagnosis.

Medullary Cystic Disease

Medullary cystic disease (ADMCKD) is a rare congenital tubulointerstitial disease associated with multiple medullary cysts almost located along the corticomedullary junction. It is an autosomal dominant disease with heterogeneous clinical manifestations and age of onset. Progression to CKD stage 5 generally occurs in patients aged around 50 years. This large clinical variability makes it very difficult to differentiate ADMCKD from other diseases as NPH or medullary sponge kidney [1, 19]. Molecular cytogenetic studies have defined 2 different forms of ADMCKD: (1) type 1, caused by a *MCKD1* gene mutation on chromosome 1 encoding an unknown protein; (2) type 2, linked to the *MCKD2* gene mutation on chromosome 16 encoding uromodulin or Tamm–Horsfall protein.

ADMCKD diagnosis is primarily based on clinical signs and family history. US diagnosis is based on the presence of small diameter junctional medullary cysts. This US finding supports the clinical suspicion but diagnosis remains undetermined without tubular function assessment and DNA sequencing. B-Mode US can highlight either normal renal volume and morphology or small kidneys with multiple cysts with a diameter (<3 cm) in the corticomedullary junction. Renal parenchyma may be normal or diffusely hyperechoic as in interstitial diseases, with widespread small microspots (fig. 5). MRI should be recommended when US is not conclusive [20].

NPH is due to a disorder of fibrocystin function, a protein of primary cilia [21]. Unlike ADMCKD, NPH is an autosomal recessive hereditary disorder that leads to end-stage renal disease during adolescence. DNA sequencing of patients and families with NPH has allowed the discovery of 8 mutations of genes encoding nephrocystin. These mutations cause ciliary dysfunction and favour the genesis of small medullary cysts (often absent in the early stages of the disease); so NPH can be confused with acquired cystic kidney disease (ACKD). Papillary microcalcifications secondary to distal tubular acidosis are very frequent in NPH. They are small calcium phosphate concretions in Bellini dilated ducts. Papillary microcalcifications can appear as renal stones with twinkling and posterior shadowing. Involvement of renal papillae may be unilateral, bilateral, segmental or diffuse. In US, renal papillae structural aspect is highly variable; it may appear normal with hypoechoic homogeneous structure if compared to the cortex or it may show an irregular structure with microvacuoles. Renal papilla features are not easily distinguishable with low frequency probes (3.5 MHz); so they must be searched using high frequencies (8 MHz) and coronal sided scans in order to reduce kidneys depth in US field of view.

ADMCKD most common form (interstitial fibrosis and tubular basement membrane thickening) is often confused with NPH. The main differences between

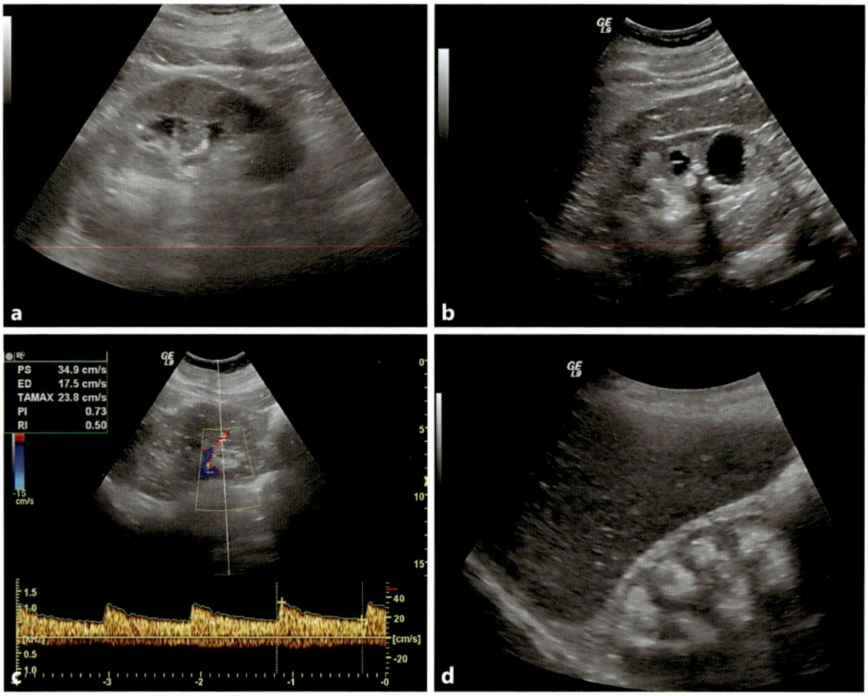

Fig. 5. ADMCKD. US can show a normal renal morphology or deformity of pyramids and papillae. **a**, **b** Medulla appears disrupted, and hypoechoic with papillary microcalcifications (Randall's plaques) and some rare medullary microcysts. **c** Doppler sampling shows normal RIs. **d** In some cases, ADMCKD morphological feature is that of nephrocalcinosis with lithiasis.

NPH and ADMCKD are (1) inheritance patterns, (2) age of onset and (3) faster progression to end-stage renal disease in NPH [22]. Differential diagnosis between NPH and ADMCKD is based on medical history, medullary cysts localization and size, absence of nephrocalcinosis and presence of calcified plaques.

Acquired Cystic Disease

ACKD results from structural end-stage kidney rearrangement and it is characterized by the presence of several small cysts without a positive history of hereditary/congenital cystic diseases [23]. Both end-stage kidneys are affected by ACKD, regardless the glomerulus tubular or ischemic origin of CKD. When GFR is 30–40 ml/min, ACKD is almost characterized by the presence of small parenchymal cysts (fig. 6) [24]. Patients with ACKD need a careful follow-up during dialysis and in the post-transplant period, because immunosuppressive therapy may be another risk factor for the onset of cancer on native kidneys.

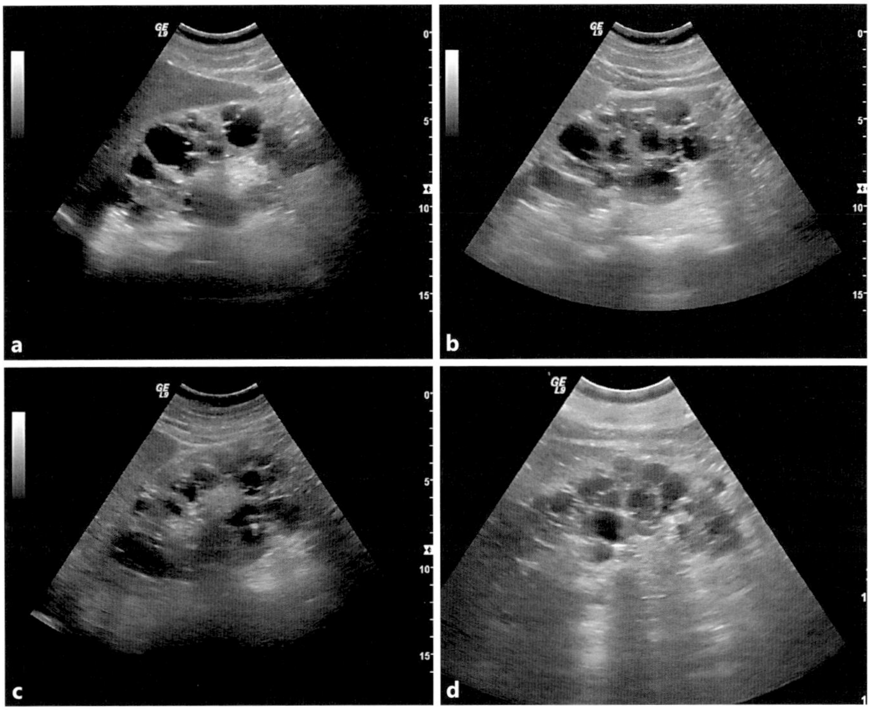

Fig. 6. ACKD. Cysts develop when glomerular filtration rate is reduced <40 ml/min and cystic degeneration progresses until end-stage renal disease. Cysts are almost small, non-confluent and have an anechoic content. In some dialysis patients, cystic degeneration can be so important that ACKD becomes indistinguishable from ADPKD. **a–d** In this case, the number of cysts is high and kidneys are increased in volume. Unlike ADPKD, cysts have a uniform diameter and are almost small (diameter <2 cm).

Conclusion

Cysts are frequently found in CKD and they may be simple solitary parenchymal cysts with no clinical significance or secondary to inherited diseases as ADPKD, ARPKD and ADMCKD. At US, simple cyst appears as a round anechoic pouch with regular and thin profiles, while in ADPKD and ARPKD kidneys show a diffuse cystic degeneration with cysts of different diameters. US evaluation of cysts is very sensitive and specific, and it allows classifying them into simple or complex cysts. This classification leads to second level imaging evaluation or to US follow-up. In ACKD, finally, US is useful not only in disease diagnosis and follow-up but also in the early detection of most severe complications, such as RCC.

References

1 Bisceglia M, Galliani CA, Senger C, Stallone C, Sessa A: Renal cystic diseases: a review. Adv Anat Pathol 2006;13:26–56.
2 Barr MM: Caenorhabditis elegans as a model to study renal development and disease: sexy cilia. J Am Soc Nephrol 2005;16:305–312.
3 Bosniak MA: The current radiological approach to renal cysts. Radiology 1986;158:1–10.
4 Schmidt T, Hohl C, Haage P, et al: Diagnostic accuracy of phase-inversion tissue harmonic imaging versus fundamental B-mode sonography in the evaluation of focal lesions of the kidney. AJR Am J Roentgenol 2003;180:1639–1647.
5 Bonsib SM: Renal cystic diseases and renal neoplasms: a mini-review. Clin J Am Soc Nephrol 2009;4:1998–2007.
6 Hartman DS, Aronson S, Frazer H: Current status of imaging indeterminate renal masses. Radiol Clin North Am 1991;29:475–496.
7 Kocaoglu M, Bulakbasi N, Ilica T, Somuncu I: MRI findings of renal lymphangiectasia. J Magn Reson Imaging 2005;22:681–683.
8 Rha SE, Byun JY, Jung SE, et al: The renal sinus: pathologic spectrum and multimodality imaging approach. Radiographics 2004;24(suppl 1):S117–S131.
9 Kazam E: Parapelvic cyst vs. hydronephrosis on coronal sonography. J Ultrasound Med 1986;5:355–356.
10 Horie S: ADPKD: molecular characterization and quest for treatment. Clin Exp Nephrol 2005;9:282–291.
11 Freire M, Remer EM: Clinical and radiologic features of cystic renal masses. AJR Am J Roentgenol 2009;192:1367–1372.
12 Pei Y, Obaji J, Dupuis A, et al: Unified criteria for ultrasonographic diagnosis of ADPKD. J Am Soc Nephrol 2009;20:205–212.
13 Fick GM, Johnson AM, Hammond WS, Gabow PA: Causes of death in autosomal dominant polycystic kidney disease. J Am Soc Nephrol 1994;24:181–187.
14 Chapman AB, Johnson AM, Rainguet S, et al: Left ventricular hypertrophy in autosomal dominant polycystic kidney disease. J Am Soc Nephrol 1997;8:1292–1297.
15 Ryu SJ: Intracranial hemorrhage in patients with polycystic kidney disease. Stroke 1990;21:291–294.
16 Torres VE, Wilson DM, Hattery RR, Segura JW: Renal stone disease in autosomal dominant polycystic kidney disease. Am J Kidney Dis 1993;22:513–519.
17 Vni FE, Guissard G, Hall M, et al: Hereditary polycystic kidney diseases in children: changing sonographic patterns through childhood. Pediatr Radiol 2002;32:169–174.
18 Blickman JG, Bramson RT, Herrin JT: Autosomal recessive polycystic kidney disease: long-term sonographic findings in patients surviving the neonatal period. AJR Am J Roentgenol 1995;164:1247–1250.
19 Wilson PD, Goilav B: Cystic disease of the kidney. Annu Rev Pathol 2007;2:341–368.
20 Meier P, Farres MT, Mougenot B, et al: Imaging medullary cystic kidney disease with magnetic resonance. Am J Kidney Dis 2003;42:E5–E10.
21 Caliskan Y, Gharavi AG: Working out nephronophthisis genetics one family at a time. J Am Soc Nephrol 2013;24:865–868.
22 Neumann HP, Zäuner I, Strahm B, et al: Late occurrence of cysts in autosomal dominant medullary cystic kidney disease. Nephrol Dial Transplant 1997;12:1242–1246.
23 Dunnill MS, Millard PR, Oliver D: Acquired cystic disease of the kidneys: a hazard of long-term intermittent maintenance haemodialysis. J Clin Pathol 1977;30:868–877.
24 Dwarakanathan S: Acquired renal cystic disease. Nephrology 2003;8:A62–A63.

Mario Meola, MD, PhD
Department of Internal Medicine
Sant'Anna School of Advanced Studies, University of Pisa
Via Savi 10, IT–56126 Pisa (Italy)
E-Mail mario.meola@unipi.it; m.meola@sssup.it

Meola M, Petrucci I, Ronco C (eds): Ultrasound Imaging in Acute and Chronic Kidney Disease.
Contrib Nephrol. Basel, Karger, 2016, vol 188, pp 131–143 (DOI: 10.1159/000445475)

Clinical Scenarios in Chronic Kidney Disease: Kidneys' Structural Changes in End-Stage Renal Disease

Mario Meola[a, b] · Sara Samoni[a, c] · Ilaria Petrucci[a, b]

[a]Sant'Anna School of Advanced Studies, Pisa, [b]Department of Internal Medicine, University of Pisa, Pisa, and [c]Department of Nephrology Dialysis and Transplantation, International Renal Research Institute (IRRIV), San Bortolo Hospital, Vicenza, Italy

Abstract

Acquired cystic kidney disease (ACKD) and renal cell carcinoma (RCC) are the most important manifestations of end-stage kidneys' structural changes. ACKD is caused by kidney damage or scarring and it is characterized by the presence of small, multiple cortical and medullary cysts filled with a fluid similar to preurine. ACKD prevalence varies according to predialysis and dialysis age and its pathogenesis is unknown, although it is stated that progressive destruction of renal tissue induces hypertrophy/compensatory hyperplasia of residual nephrons and may trigger the degenerative process. ACKD is almost asymptomatic, but it can lead to several complications (bleeding, rupture, infections, RCC). Ultrasound (US) is the first level imaging technique in ACKD, because of its sensitivity and reliability. The most serious complication of ACKD is RCC, which is stimulated by the same growth factors and proto-oncogenes that lead to the genesis of cysts. Two different histological types of RCC have been identified: (1) RCC associated with ACKD and (2) papillary renal clear cell carcinoma. Tumors in end-stage kidneys are mainly small, multifocal and bilateral, with a papillary structure and a low degree of malignancy. At US, RCC appears as a small inhomogeneous nodule (<3 cm), clearly outlined from the renal profile and hypoechoic if compared with sclerotic parenchyma. In some cases, tumor appears as a homogeneous and hyperechoic multifocal mass. The most specific US sign of a small tumor in end-stage kidney is the important arterial vascularization, in contrast with renal parenchymal vascular sclerosis.

Acquired Cystic Kidney Disease

Epidemiology

Acquired cystic kidney disease (ACKD) is caused by kidney damage or scarring. ACKD is characterized by the presence of small, multiple cortical and medullary cysts (at least 3 in each kidney), filled with a fluid similar to preurine (fig. 1). ACKD in chronic dialysis patients has been reported for the first time in the 1970s [1]. In the following years, several studies have confirmed the first observations and have also demonstrated the relationship between ACKD and renal cell carcinoma (RCC) [2]. Cysts begin to form when glomerular filtration rate (GFR) is <30–40 ml/min; so, approximately 8–22% of patients with chronic kidney disease (CKD) have ACKD before starting dialysis [3]. In dialysis, ACKD prevalence varies according to dialytic age [4] and it affects 13%, 50% and 87% of patients after 2, 6 and 9 years of dialysis, respectively, and almost 100% of patients after 10 years [5]. ACKD progression slows after 10–15 years of dialysis. ACKD is less common in peritoneal patients and regresses after transplantation [6]. However, many native kidneys continue to form cysts after renal transplantation if renal function remains impaired. ACKD is more common in men (prevalence 3:1) and does not correlate with age, race, dialysis technique and CKD etiology [7]. At autopsy, kidneys appear structureless, reduced in volume and contain many cysts of different diameter. At histology, cyst wall is made of a single layer of epithelial cubic or flattened cells and, in 60% of cases, it shows hyperplastic and dysplastic degeneration with proliferative papillary or adeno-papillary aspects [1, 5]. Cysts almost contain a turbid liquid chemically similar to preurine often mixed with calcium oxalate crystals, blood catabolites, cytokines and growth factors. Atypical epithelial cell clusters, low-grade malignant carcinomatous cells or isolated benign epithelial cells can be depicted in the sediment of complicated or complex cysts [8].

Pathogenesis of ACKD

ACKD pathogenesis is unknown, although it is stated that progressive destruction of renal tissue induces hypertrophy/compensatory hyperplasia of residual nephrons and may trigger the degenerative process. Pathogenetic mechanisms responsible of cysts formation are (1) tubular obstruction, (2) expression of growth factors and proto-oncogenes and (3) ischemia. The first hypothesis is that tubular obstruction, caused by precipitation of crystals of calcium oxalate and interstitial fibrosis, favors cysts formation. Intracystic fluid accumulation would result from residual glomerular filtration and tubular secretion. The second hypothesis is that hypertrophy/hyperplasia of tubular epithelium (activated

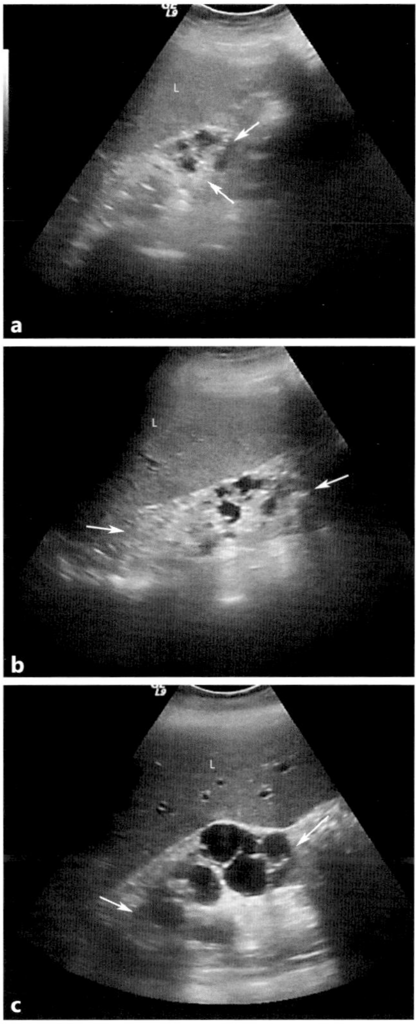

Fig. 1. Kidneys' structural changes in end stage renal disease. The presence of small, multiple, cortical and medullary fluid-filled cysts (at least 3 in each kidney) characterizes the ACKD (**a–c**). Sometimes, only the presence of cysts helps to identify an atrophic kidney, often poorly recognizable in the retroperitoneum (white arrows). L = Liver.

by mitogenic factors such as electrolyte imbalance and decreased excretion of H^+) leads to an increased expression of growth factors and activation of proto-oncogenes as c-ERB_2. Growth factors may favor the formation of cysts in association with an increased transepithelial secretion supported by increased levels of PTH and other factors such as secretin, vasoactive intestinal peptide and high levels of vasopressin [3, 4, 7]. Ischemic hypothesis is derived from the observation that clinical ACKD is a common occurrence in end-stage ischemic nephropathy secondary to main artery stenosis and/or nephroangiosclerosis. Cysts development is induced by tubular cells necrosis, tubular obstruction, acidosis and release of cytokines and growth factors, even when renal artery obstruction is secondary to end-stage renal disease [9].

Clinical Signs and Complications

ACKD is almost asymptomatic but it can lead to several complications. In 15% of cases, bleeding or rupture of one or more cysts may complicate ACKD. This event causes intense sharp flank pain and may be associated with hematuria. The rupture of one or more cysts can lead to a perirenal or retroperitoneal spontaneous hematoma and, when bleeding is severe, it can cause a hypovolemic shock (Wunderlich syndrome). Dystrophic cystic calcifications are almost consequent to parietal remodelling secondary to bleeding. Infection that leads to renal/pararenal abscess with sepsis is a rare complication. It is even rarer to diagnose erythrocytosis due to erythropoietin hypersecretion in ACKD patients. Exceptionally, the finding of metastatic RCC represents the onset of ACKD.

The risk of RCC is over 40 times higher in end-stage ACKD than it is in general population and it represents the most severe complication. The prevalence of RCC in native kidneys after transplantation is approximately 5%, in ACKD hemodialysis patients is about 19% and in patients with complex cysts is 54%. Papillary carcinoma is the most common histological type in ACKD. Tumor is multicentric in at least 50% of cases and bilateral in 10% of cases [10].

Imaging

Ultrasound (US) is the first level imaging technique in ACKD, because of its sensitivity and reliability. At US, kidneys appear structureless and hyperechoic with irregular profiles. Small parenchymal cysts <3 cm are diffused in both kidneys (fig. 2). Sometimes, after long dialytic periods, acquired cystic degeneration is so massive that it is difficult to differentiate ACKD from polycystic disease [4]. The most important differential criteria are the absence of inheritance and family history of cystic disease and, vice versa, a history of renal parenchymal disease. Morphological parameters that allow the differential diagnosis between ACKD and polycystic kidney disease (PKD) are kidney size and the absence of cysts in other organs such as liver, pancreas and ovary. In PKD, parenchyma is unrecognizable because of cystic massive degeneration. The number of renal cysts is so high that is impossible to count them and kidney is so increased in volume that it occupies the lumbar fossa, the pelvis and the median retroperitoneum. In ACKD, kidneys are small, structureless, with small parenchymal residues and a small number of cysts. Sometimes, cysts may have a complex morphology or a corpuscular/partially solid content. Differential diagnosis between small complex cysts and small adenomas can be very difficult because of partial volume artifact. In any case, from a clinical point of view, the problem should not be overestimated. In fact, most postmortem histological examinations confirm the association between ACKD

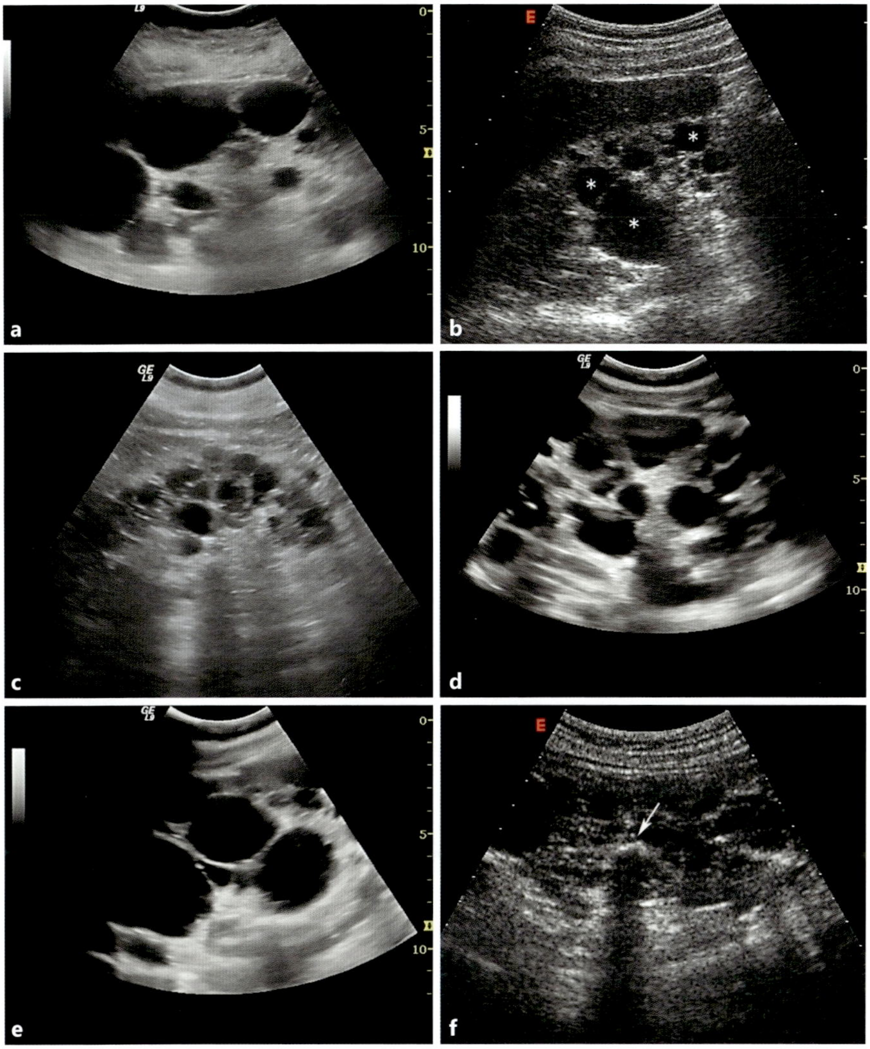

Fig. 2. Kidneys' structural changes in end-stage renal disease. **a–e** Cysts number, distribution and morphology (*) are variable and depend on the time of uremia. Typically the diameter is <2–3 cm. **f** Calcifications (white arrow) or nephrocalcinosis can be present in ACKD.

and abnormal proliferative lesions within the cysts in about 60% of patients, without any evidence of cancer [1]. However, it is important to identify larger solid lesions, which can be a malignant neoplasm. In summary, ACKD diagnosis during predialysis is easy to perform because (1) cysts are few, (2) cysts develop as CKD progresses, (3) renal parenchyma between cysts shows a normal structure and (4) patient's clinical history does not reveal any hereditary/

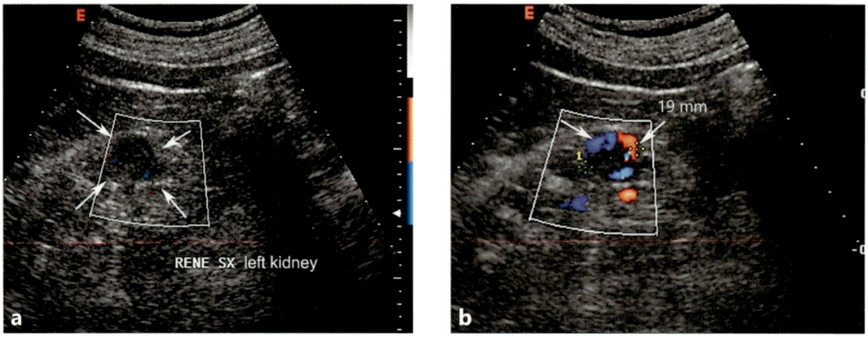

Fig. 3. ACKD and RCC. RCC in ACKD often appears as an exophytic, solid, hyperechoic and small nodule. Therefore it can be easily misdiagnosed in the context of an atrophic kidney (**a**). Color Doppler sampling shows a rich vascularization (**b**), incompatible with typical sclerofibrosis of residual renal parenchyma, thus helping the diagnosis of RCC.

congenital cystic disease, but it highlights a chronic parenchymal disease. In dialysis patients, ACKD can rapidly worsen and the kidney structure that has already been altered by chronic parenchymal disease is almost represented by multiple cysts <3 cm. There can be so many cysts that it becomes difficult to differentiate ACKD from adult dominant PKD. Clinical and family history allows an immediate differential diagnosis.

At color Doppler, cysts show no signs of wall perfusion. The presence of a perfused solid nodule in the context of an end-stage kidney is an almost indicative sign of malignancy (fig. 3). In these cases, contrast-enhanced ultrasound (CEUS) imaging should be performed before contrast-enhanced computed tomography (CT) and magnetic resonance imaging (MRI). In current clinical practice, CT and MRI are used for follow-up and for complications, while US is extensively used for screening of dialysis patients. US is indicated in the screening of complex cysts because it is more sensitive than CT without contrast media as small hemorrhagic cysts appear to be iso-dense or slightly hyperdense [11, 12]. CEUS is very useful in differential diagnosis although there are few specific studies. MRI may instead be very useful in differentiating infected or bleeding cysts from cystic kidney cancer [13]. ACKD complications are bleeding, infection, ureteral stones and kidney tumors. Intracystic bleeding is common and it is asymptomatic in approximately 50% of patients [14]. Severe bleeding with cyst rupture may instead cause a perirenal or retroperitoneal severe hematoma.

ACKD patients require a careful follow-up either in dialysis or in the post-transplant period when immunosuppressive therapy may be another risk factor for the onset of cancer on native kidneys. After transplantation, the prevalence of cancer in native kidneys is approximately 5%, in hemodialysis ACKD patients

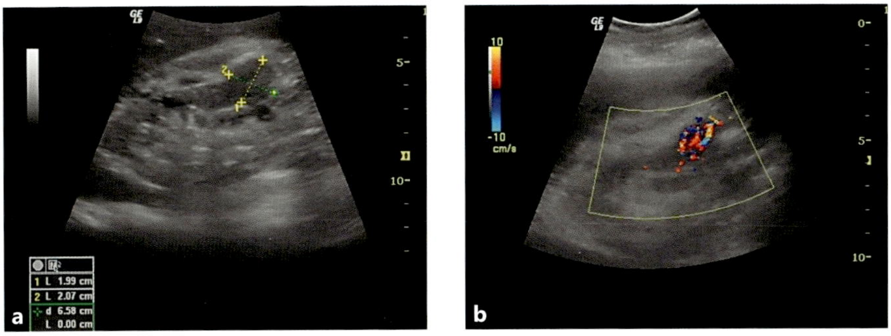

Fig. 4. Patient with kidney transplant and RCC of native kidney. Male, aged 73 years, with a histological diagnosis of interstitial nephropathy, in hemodialysis from 1995 to 1997. Kidney transplant in 1997. In 2012, serum creatinine was 3.2 mg/dl and creatinine clearance 19 ml/min. **a** The right native kidney shows a small isoechoic nodule well outlined from the lower renal pole. **b** Color Doppler shows a rich vascularization within the nodule, while the renal atrophic parenchyma is not vascularized.

is 19% and in patients with complex cysts is 54%. These data suggest that transplanted patients need an accurate follow-up once a year in order to exclude neoplasms in native kidneys [15]. The 5-year survival after diagnosis of renal cancer is comparable with that observed in the general population [16].

Renal Cell Carcinoma

Prevalence and Physiopathology

The most serious complication of ACKD is RCC, which is stimulated by the same growth factors and proto-oncogenes that lead to the genesis of cysts. It affects 5% of dialysis patients [17], is more common in men (prevalence 7:1) and can develop even after transplant. Two different histological types of RCC have been identified: (1) RCC associated with ACKD and (2) papillary renal clear cell carcinoma. RCC associated with ACKD shows a more aggressive histology; it requires surgery, but it is a rare cause of death in dialysis patients. The prevalence of RCC requires annual monitoring in patients undergoing transplantation and in dialysis patients. In transplanted patients, native kidney tumors have a more aggressive behavior and can metastasize because of immunosuppressive therapy (fig. 4) [18]. Cancer is one of the leading causes of long-term mortality in transplanted patients [19]. Therefore, despite the low prevalence and the reduced risk of RCC due to the use of new immunosuppressive drugs, some authors propose an active surveillance of native kidneys in pre-transplant or transplanted patients [15].

Several studies have compared the biological characteristics of sporadic kidney cancer and of cancer in end-stage kidneys with ACKD. Tumors in end-stage kidneys are mainly small, multifocal and bilateral, with a papillary structure and a low degree of malignancy. In addition, they are less aggressive and have a survival rate at 5 years greater than sporadic tumors. These data, nevertheless, should be carefully considered. In a recent observational study that has analysed the tumor doubling time, it was observed that end-stage kidney cancer shows a growth rate of 0.5–1 cm/year in 75% of cases and a faster growth rate, ≥6 cm/year, in 25% of cases [20]. These data demonstrate that epithelial tumors that develop in end-stage kidneys have a great heterogeneity. However, ACKD is not a prerequisite for the development of cancer in end-stage kidneys and it represents, as carcinoma, the result of a structural rearrangement of end-stage parenchyma. From a histological point of view, end-stage kidney cancer may have its own biological characteristics or may be similar to sporadic tumors. A first histological type (carcinoma in ACKD) is a tumor that shows eosinophilic cells arranged in tubulocystic architecture [21]. This histological structure is not exclusive of carcinoma in ACKD, but it is characteristic for the presence of several intracellular birefringent crystals of calcium oxalate. The second type of recurrent tumor in end-stage kidneys is the papillary clear cell carcinoma, similar to sporadic cancer, but with a papillary structural arrangement. Metastases are very rare in the first histological type and they have never been reported in papillary clear cell carcinoma [22].

Imaging

US diagnosis of end-stage kidney tumor requires a skilled operator on US since end-stage kidneys are small (<5–6 cm), fibrosclerotic and hardly distinguishable into the retroperitoneal space. Small acquired cysts can help in identifying end-stage kidney. Kidney profiles and sinus structures are unrecognizable.

At US, RCC appears as a small inhomogeneous nodule (<3 cm), clearly outlined from the renal profile and hypoechoic if compared with sclerotic parenchyma (fig. 5). In some cases, tumor appears as a homogeneous and hyperechoic multifocal mass. This commonly occurs in adenomatous nodules associated with chronic reflux nephropathy. The most specific US sign of a small tumor in end-stage kidney is the important arterial vascularization (peak systolic velocity >30 cm/s), which contrasts with renal parenchyma diffused vascular sclerosis. Parenchymal and vascular structure of small tumors can be better characterized with US 3-dimensional (3D) imaging (fig. 6). CEUS utility is unknown due to few data in literature. CT or MRI should complete RCC diagnosis with contrast medium, especially in pseudocystic tumors

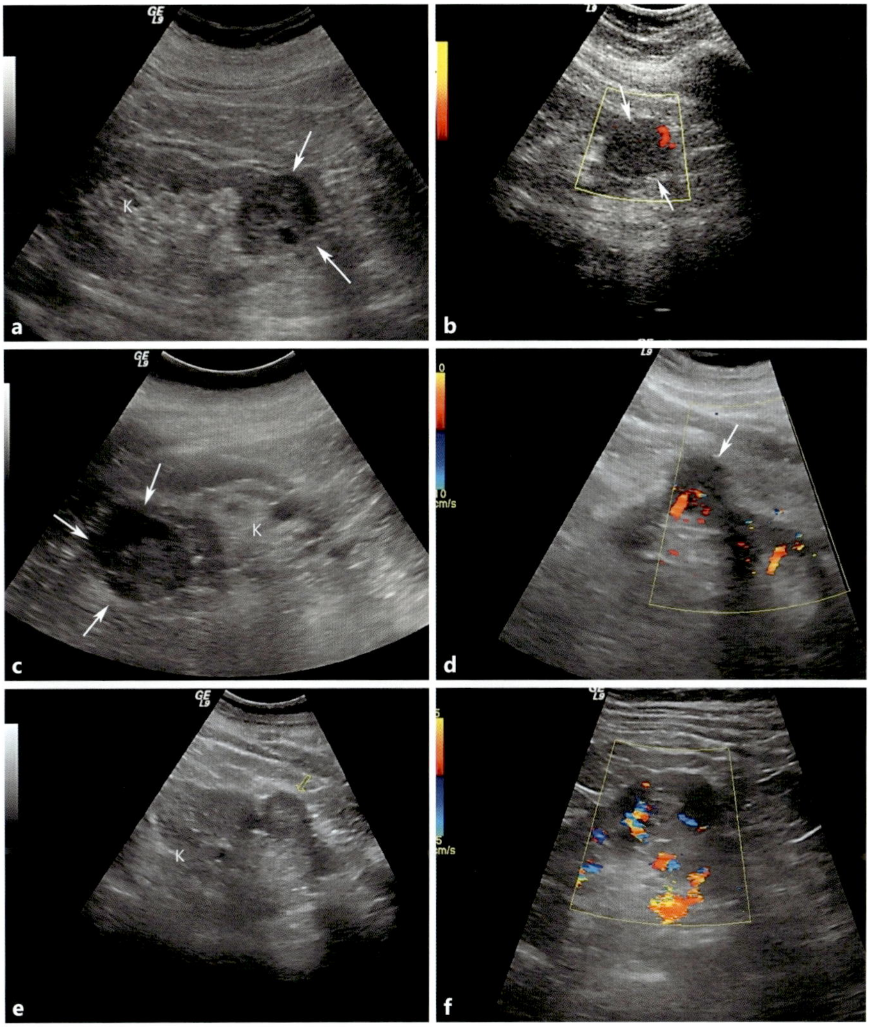

Fig. 5. RCC in end-stage kidney. CKD stage 4. **a** Small hypoechoic nodule deforming the parenchymal profile, which is thinned and sclerotic. **b** Renal nodule shows a poor peripheral vascularization. **c** CKD stage 5. RCC in end-stage kidney. Exophytic lesion is well evident because it alters kidney profile and appears hypervascularized (**d**). **e**, **f** CKD stage 5. Carcinoma of end-stage kidney <3 cm, with inhomogeneous feature and irregular vascularization. K = Kidney.

(fig. 7), in order to distinguish between complex hemorragic cysts and small cystic tumors. Guidelines state that US should be performed every year for cancer screening in dialysis and transplanted patients. US is needed to evaluate the cancer growth rate in those cases in which active surveillance is to be preferred over surgical excision [15].

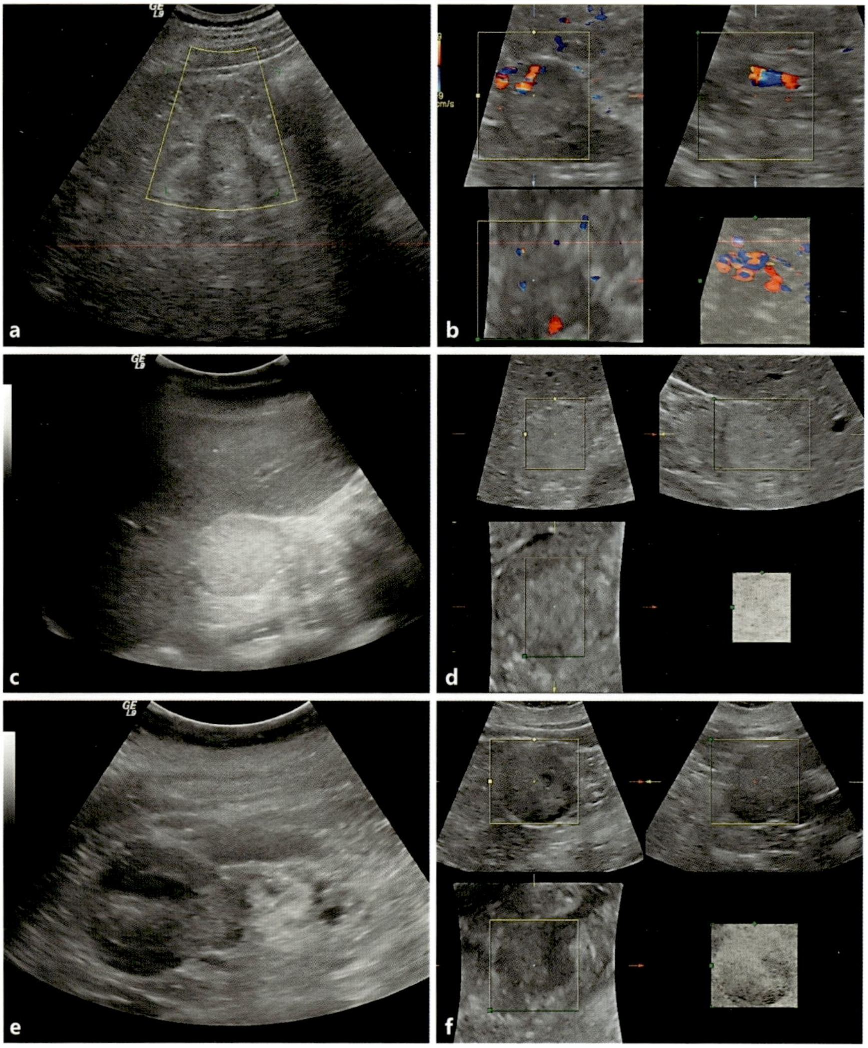

Fig. 6. RCC in end-stage kidney with ACKD. Three different cases of kidney cancer in end-stage kidney with ACKD have been studied with a 3-dimensional (3D) volumetric probe. 3D analysis can help to better study tumor vascularization (**a**, **b**), or its morphology in the 3 planes and in volume rendering. **c** Solid homogenous and hyperechoic neoplasm in end-stage kidney (histological diagnosis of renal adenoma). **d** Volumetric reconstruction. **e** Tumor necrotic component. Conventional scan (**e**) and 3D volume acquisition (**f**).

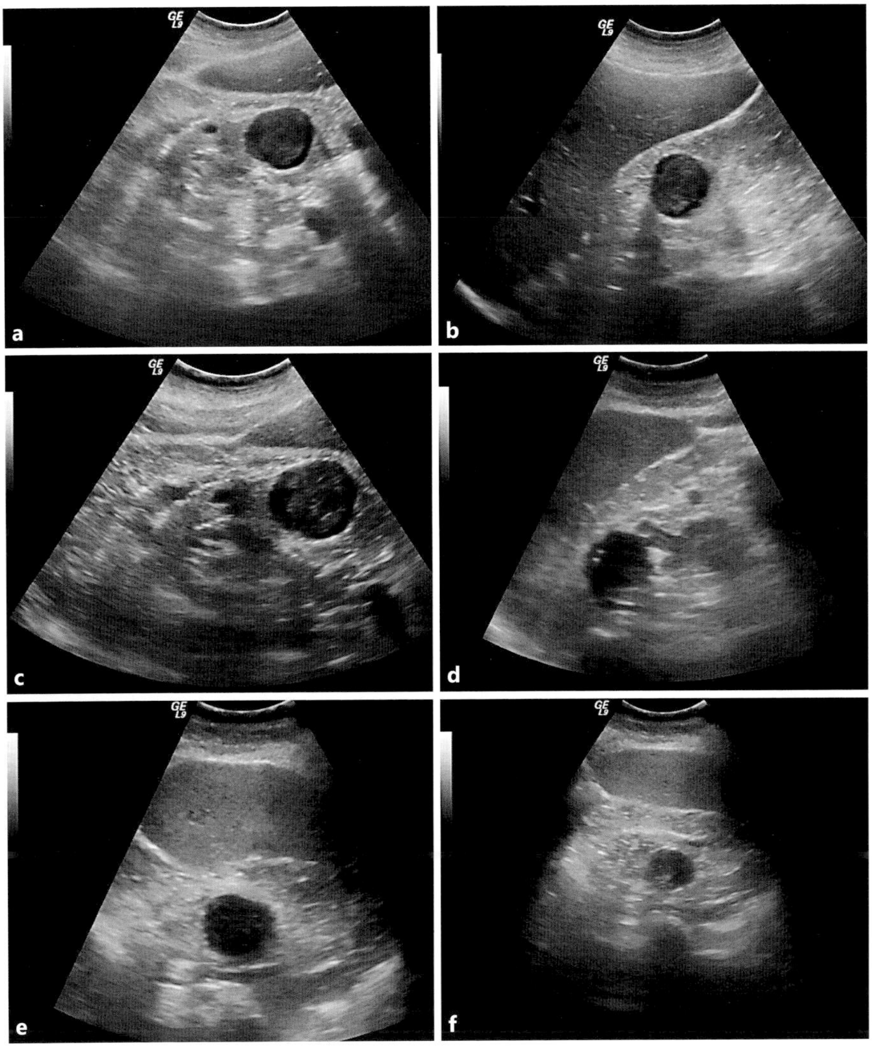

Fig. 7. RCC in end-stage kidney. US diagnosis of RCC must be confirmed by contrast-enhanced CT or MRI, especially in cystic forms. **a–c** Cystic tumor confirmed by CT. **d–f** A cystic form of RCC was suspected at US, instead MRI has diagnosed a complicated cyst.

Conclusion

ACKD and RCC are the most important manifestations of end-stage kidney structural changes. US is the first level imaging technique in ACKD, because of its sensitivity and reliability. Patients with ACKD, either in pre-dialysis/dialysis or in transplant period, have to be carefully followed-up in order to exclude the presence of the most serious complication of ACKD, that is, RCC. At US, RCC appears as a small inhomogeneous nodule (<3 cm), clearly outlined from the renal profile and hypoechoic if compared with sclerotic parenchyma. In some cases, tumor appears as a homogeneous and hyperechoic multifocal mass. The most specific US sign of a small tumor in end-stage kidney is the important arterial vascularization, which contrasts with renal parenchyma diffused vascular sclerosis.

References

1 Dunnill MS, Millard PR, Oliver D: Acquired cystic disease of the kidneys: a hazard of long-term intermittent maintenance haemodialysis. J Clin Pathol 1977;30:868–877.
2 Oya M, Mikami S, Mizuno R, Marumo K, Mukai M, Murai M: C-jun activation in acquired cystic kidney disease and renal cell carcinoma. J Urol 2005;174:726.
3 Grantham JJ: Acquired cystic kidney disease. Kidney Int 1991;40:143–152.
4 Levine E: Acquired cystic kidney disease. Radiol Clin North Am 1996;34:947–964.
5 Truong LD, Choi YJ, Shen SS, Ayala G, Amato R, Krishnan B: Renal cystic neoplasms and renal neoplasms associated with cystic renal diseases: pathogenetic and molecular links. Adv Anat Pathol 2003;10:135–159.
6 Lien YH, Hunt KR, Siskind MS, Zukoski C: Association of cyclosporin A with acquired cystic kidney disease of the native kidneys in renal transplant recipients. Kidney Int 1993; 44:613–616.
7 Nahm AM, Ritz E: Acquired renal cysts. Nephrol Dial Transplant 2001;16:1506–1508.
8 Todd TD, Dhurandhar B, Mody D, Ramzy I, Truong LD: Fine-needle aspiration of cystic lesions of the kidney. Morphologic spectrum and diagnostic problems in 41 cases. Am J Clin Pathol 1999;111:317–328.
9 Cohen EP, Elliott WC Jr: The role of ischemia in acquired cystic kidney disease. Am J Kidney Dis 1990;15:55–60.
10 Kuroda N, Ohe C, Mikami S, Hes O, Michal M, Brunelli M, et al: Review of acquired cystic disease-associated renal cell carcinoma with focus on pathobiological aspects. Histol Histopathol 2011;26:1215–1218.
11 Paudice N, Zanazzi M, Agostini S, Bertelli E, Caroti L, Carta P, et al: Contrast-enhanced ultrasound assessment of complex cystic lesions in renal transplant recipients with acquired cystic kidney disease: preliminary experience. Transplant Proc 2012;44: 1928–1929.
12 Rule AD, Sasiwimonphan K, Lieske JC, Keddis MT, Torres VE, Vrtiska TJ: Characteristics of renal cystic and solid lesions based on contrast-enhanced computed tomography of potential kidney donors. Am J Kidney Dis 2012;59:611–618.
13 Takase Y, Kodama K, Motoi I, Saito K: Cyst infection in unilateral renal cystic disease and the role of diffusion-weighted magnetic resonance imaging. Urology 2012;80:e61–e62.
14 Ishikawa I: Hemorrhage versus cancer in acquired cystic disease. Semin Dial 2000;13:56.
15 Scandling JD: Acquired cystic kidney disease and renal cell cancer after transplantation: time to rethink screening? Clin J Am Soc Nephrol 2007;2:621–622.
16 Webster WS, Thompson RH, Cheville JC, Lohse CM, Blute ML, Leibovich BC: Surgical resection provides excellent outcomes for patients with cystic clear cell renal cell carcinoma. Urology 2007;70:900–904; discussion 904.
17 Stewart JH, Buccianti G, Agodoa L, et al: Cancers of the kidney and urinary tract in patients on dialysis for end-stage renal disease: analysis of data from the United States, Europe, and Australia and New Zealand. J Am Soc Nephrol 2003;14:197–207.
18 Schwarz A, Vatandaslar S, Merkel S, Haller H: Renal cell carcinoma in transplant recipients with acquired cystic kidney disease. Clin J Am Soc Nephrol 2007;2:750–756.

19 Dantal J, Pohanka E: Malignancies in renal transplantation: an unmet medical need. Nephrol Dial Transplant 2007;22(suppl 1):i4–i10.

20 Takebayashi S, Hidai H, Chiba T, Irisawa M, Matsubara S: Renal cell carcinoma in acquired cystic kidney disease: volume growth rate determined by helical computed tomography. Am J Kidney Dis 2000;36:759–766.

21 Tickoo SK, DePeralta-Venturina MN, Harik LR, Worcester HD, Salama M, Young AN, Moch H, Amin MB: Spectrum of epithelial neoplasms in end-stage renal disease. An experience for 66 tumor-bearing kidneys with emphasis on histologic patterns distinct form those in sporadic adult renal neoplasia. Am J Surg Pathol 2006;30:141–153.

22 Nguyen MM, Gill IS: Effect of renal cancer size on the prevalence of metastasis at diagnosis and mortality. J Urol 2009;181:1020–1027; discussion 1027.

Mario Meola, MD, PhD
Department of Internal Medicine
Sant'Anna School of Advanced Studies, University of Pisa
Via Savi 10, IT–56126 Pisa (Italy)
E-Mail mario.meola@unipi.it; m.meola@sssup.it

Author Index

Subject Index